HORMONE REPLACEMENT THERAPIES:

Astonishing Results for Men and Women

William Campbell Douglass, MD

Rhino Publishing, S.A.

HORMONE REPLACEMENT THERAPIES:

Astonishing Results for Men and Women

ISBN 9962-636-22-1

Cover illustration by

Alex Manyoma (alex@3dcity.com)

Please, visit Rhino's website for other publications from Dr. William Campbell Douglass
www.rhinopublish.com

Dr. Douglass' "Real Health" alternative medical newsletter is available at www.realhealthnews.com

RHINO PUBLISHING, S.A.
World Trade Center
Panama, Republic of Panama

Voicemail/Fax
International: + 416-352-5126
North America: 888-317-6767

Contents

HORMONE REPLACEMENT THERAPIES: ASTONISHING RESULTS FOR MEN AND WOMEN

Pat Kay had been a circus performer. She had beautiful red hair and rode horses in the show. She showed me pictures of her when she was 20 and in her costume — a living doll of about 100 pounds. When I met her as a patient, she weighed 220.

"I know why my weight suddenly increased," she said, "but no one will believe me." She and her husband were involved in a serious automobile accident in which she suffered a serious head injury and was in a coma for a week.

"After that," she said, "my weight started increasing and has never stopped. Something happened in my head."

She developed diabetes, hypertension, severe fluid retention, complete cessation of her periods, myxedema (thyroid dysfunction), adrenal dysfunction, and many other problems that would indicate a *severely damaged pituitary gland.*

I told her that the connection between the head injury and the accident was so dramatic that I had to believe her. But that was back in 1962 and I knew I was not qualified to handle such a complicated hormonal case. I sent her to an endocrinologist who said the head injury couldn't cause her condition and that her problem was neurosis — so he sent her to a psychiatrist. She died of heart failure at the age of 45.

Fortunately, not all hormone cases are this drastic, but the problems are no less troublesome. The medical profession has known of hormone therapy for 40 years, but it's still gone unused. Why? The reasons most of the hormones discussed in this monograph don't get to you for the improvement of your health and increased longevity are politics and money, with a little doctor ignorance thrown in.

Hormones are "chemical messengers," the bureaucrats in your body who run the whole show, you might say. The term was invented in 1904 to describe the secretions that had been discovered to come from certain glands, such as the thyroid and the pituitary, that had a heretofore unknown way of entering into the regulation of the body. These researchers found that the glands secrete the chemical *directly into the bloodstream,* rather than squirt it into a hollow space, such as from the lining of the stomach into the stomach cavity.

These glands without any visible means of delivery of its secretions were called endocrine glands. This bloodstream delivery system was a momentous discovery from which the specialty of endocrinology developed. These glands have also been termed "ductless glands," meaning they have no passageway for the delivery of their chemicals. The gall bladder would be an example of a gland that delivers its secretions by way of a duct, or tube, into the intestinal tract.

This monograph will be about these "ductless," or endocrine, glands and how they quietly regulate your life and your health. It is accurate to say that when the endocrine glands start to fail, you start to die. What most doctors don't realize is that we are facing a sea change in longevity and health in the elderly. Now, with the proper supplemental hormones, we can slow the aging process and, in many cases, reverse some of the signs and symptoms of aging.

The Little Gland That Could

Our redheaded friend suspected something was wrong in her head, and as I said, she probably damaged her pituitary gland when she suffered the head injury. But there's another gland in the brain that has replaced the pituitary gland for the honor of being called the "master gland." It's called the pineal gland.

As you get older, the pineal shrinks dramatically, starting around age 20. With this involution, there is often a calcification of the gland and a steady decrease in hormone production — about one percent per year. Is it any wonder then that the elderly suffer from decreased sexual function, low energy levels, failing eyesight, and susceptibility to infection and degenerative diseases?

I was taught in medical school (in the mid 1950s) that the pineal "body" was some sort of leftover from evolution. The standard joke said that it was "the seat of the soul," but I never believed it. It has nerve fibers running out of it, so I figured it was more important than that.

My *Dorland's Medical Dictionary*, 20th edition, describes the pineal gland as a pine-cone-shaped "body" located at the epithalamus and an outgrowth thereof. "It is not composed of nervous (sic) elements and is a rudimentary (i.e., undeveloped) glandular structure said to produce an internal secretion." So, since I left medical school, the pineal *body* has become the pineal *gland*. It is your chief photoreceptor — a receptor of photons from the heavens to the eye and on to the pineal, which then manufactures the hormones, some known and some not yet discovered.

Well, maybe it *is* the seat of the soul, but it also protects the body from light deficiency and is now considered to be the master gland that controls all the others. So the little, insignificant pineal has gone from a "rudimentary glandular structure ... said to produce an internal secretion," to the Master Regulator of all the glands — and all this flowering has taken place during my lifetime.

But there's one problem: Calcification of the pineal gland occurs in a large percentage of people over 60 years of age. This calcification is not a "natural part of the aging process," because it doesn't happen in everyone, but it is very

7

common. As an emergency medicine specialist for 20 years, I saw many sick elderly people and the calcified pineal gland was a common finding. Before the advent of CAT scans and EMR, the gland was used as a diagnostic tool for finding a space-occupying mass in the brain. If an X ray revealed that the pineal was shifted to one side from its normal place in the midline, then you knew that something was pushing it off center, like a tumor or a blood clot.

I'm giving you this anatomy/physiology lesson because I think it has relevance to the treatment of many things that ail you. If we could decalcify, and thus rejuvenate the pineal gland, we might be able to solve a lot of medical problems. This decalcification might, in fact, be part of the reason why chelation therapy helps so many people. I wonder if anyone has ever analyzed the mineral content of the "calcified" pineal. Maybe it contains iron as well as calcium — and possibly aluminum and mercury.

A report in the journal *Lancet,* revealed that *there was a direct statistical correlation between the incidence of breast cancer and the rate of pineal calcification.* In the United States, for example, there is a high rate of pineal calcification and a high rate of breast cancer. In Japan, there is a low rate of pineal calcification and a low rate of breast cancer.

There are few areas of medicine where the hormones of this little gland do not play a role. This pea-sized structure is certainly "the little gland that could." Even cardiovascular disease, Alzheimer's disease, asthma, diabetes, and Parkinson's disease are improved with hormones from the pineal gland.

One of the most exciting areas of study is in diseases of the eye. Glaucoma, macular degeneration, and cataracts are three of the areas of medicine where the diagnoses are excellent, but the treatment often discouraging. The hormones of the pineal are going to play a major role in the treatment and prevention of these major causes of blindness, once we get it all sorted out.

So far, we've only discussed one major gland in the body. We haven't even touched on the thymus gland, the adrenal glands, and many others that produce essential hormones for healthy living. But before we can talk about the benefits of this hormone revolution, we must first debunk many of the untruths you're being told by conventional medicine.

Many of you are aware of conventional medicine's version of hormone therapy for treating osteoporosis and other ailments. But sadly, the results have been anything but rewarding. For some reason (money and politics), doctors are glad to prescribe the wrong estrogen (a drug from horse urine), the wrong progesterone (a synthetic, which isn't progesterone), and a highly destructive drug (fluoride) for osteoporosis. And yet they have prescribed little if any vitamin D, which is one of the good hormones in short supply, and they have ignored the *benefits* of testosterone for *both men and women*. These are just a few examples of the incredible neglect and mistreatment in the field of hormone therapy.

Estrogen

The most famous of the hormone replacement therapies is estrogen, which has been used for years in the treatment of osteoporosis. But you will be shocked to find out how backward American doctors are in regard to this therapy. The prescription drug is called Premarin, the synthetic "estrogen" from horse urine. But *it's not estrogen.*

Here's the description of Premarin that the company wrote for the *Physician's Desk Reference:* It "contains a mixture of estrogens obtained exclusively from natural sources ... blended to represent the average composition of material derived from pregnant mares' urine. It contains estrone, equilin, and 17 a-dihydroequilin, together with smaller amounts of 17 a-estradiol, equilenin and 17 a-dihydroequilenin...."

9

There are actually three human estrogens produced by the body. They are estradiol, estrone, and estriol. While Premarin does cause the level of estrogen in the body to increase, the body does not manufacture anything called equilin, equilenin, a-dihydroequilin, or a-dihydroequilenin. What *is* all this stuff anyway? Should you be taking it just because it's "exclusively from natural sources"? Hashish and botulinum toxin are from natural sources, so does that make them okay to take for your hot flashes?

This is just the beginning. There are now reports of women addicted to Premarin. Many women who take synthetic estrogen to prevent aging and osteoporosis are taking elephant doses to stave off these problems and are greatly increasing their chances of getting cancer of the breast. One expert on women's health, Susan Bewley of the London St. Thomas' Hospital, reports that women develop resistance to synthetic estrogen the same way that addicts develop resistance to heroin and cocaine. Some of these women have estrogen levels *10 times* that of much younger women.

Dr. Gaye Higham from the menopause clinic at Newcastle (England) General Hospital said: "We don't know what the long-term effect of high doses of circulating (synthetic) estrogen will be." Well, we *do* know the long-term effect: Studies have shown very clearly that Premarin causes an increased risk of developing *cancer.*

It has been clearly established that if Premarin works at all in the treatment of osteoporosis, and it has been used for this purpose for the past 40 years, it works *only while it is being taken.* This means that one must take the "estrogen" from menopause to death, which exposes the patient to an enormous increase in the risk of contracting breast or endometrial cancer.

Estrogen replacement therapy for osteoporosis is one of the great medical hoaxes of the 20th century. It doesn't work, except temporarily in some cases, and it greatly increases the risk of cancer. You don't have to take my word for it; read it yourself in the *American Journal of Medicine* (1988;85:847-50).

But the troubles with estrogen don't end there. Some researchers even think that estrogen replacement therapy actually *causes* osteoporosis due to tiny blood clots that form in the bone when estrogen is given experimentally to animals.

Something else the doctor doesn't tell you, because he probably doesn't know it, is that estrogen replacement therapy depresses the blood levels of alkaline phosphatase. Depressed alkaline phosphatase levels means that magnesium cannot stimulate calcium deposition in bone. So you can see that it's not so farfetched to say that *estrogen replacement therapy causes osteoporosis.*

Professor Leon Speroff of the Oregon Medical School in Portland, says he's worried about "hysteria" from women being told the truth about estrogen causing cancer. (I guess he doesn't have to worry about Dr. Higham telling anybody as, apparently, she doesn't know.) He implied, in a FedEx letter to the world, that the Harvard study was "unbalanced," whatever that means, and he "urged caution" in interpreting the work of the Harvard group that was uncomplimentary toward Premarin.

Speroff says he is "speaking independently," but, it should be noted, he has been paid for clinical trials in the past by the makers of Premarin, the billion-dollar winner in the estrogen sales business. It's sort of like working for the CIA. Once you are on the payroll, you are always on a leash and can be called back. And in the case of clinical researchers, they *want* to be called back — the pay is good and the work practically nonexistent.

Added to the problem of greed is the problem of maleducation of doctors. The maleducation, or miseducation, is impossible to avoid. In medical school, they were honest enough to warn us that half of what they were teaching us was wrong — "But we just don't know which half." This was

11

an amusing way of telling us the absolute truth. But, even having admitted this, they will react with awesome ferocity when one of those students grows up and challenges them on "the wrong half." As Arthur Koestler said in *The Age of Velikovsky*, "Innovation is a twofold threat to the scientific community. First, it threatens their oracle authority. Secondly, it evokes the deeper fear that their whole laboriously constructed authoritarian edifice may collapse."

Enough about the medical sleaze and medical holy doctrine that passes for science and on to a look on the positive side. There are over 20 drugs now in development for the treatment of osteoporosis and about half of them are not related to estrogen at all. Out of this flock of new drugs, there actually may be a real winner in the fight against osteoporosis, which in its extreme form is a terrible disease among women — and a few good men. If these new drugs are half as good as they sound, I hope the stockholders make millions. But I suggest that you wait and let them do their experimenting on someone else before taking these new pharmaceuticals. Previous experience with anti-osteoporosis drugs has not been encouraging.

Finally, the doctors and drug companies have realized that American women are no longer willing to risk cancer of the breast to prevent osteoporosis, a disease that is terrible, but at least it's not cancer. I hope the doctors succeed with these new drugs, but I remain skeptical.

If you do take estrogen, make sure the doctor understands the difference between horses and humans — many don't. Earlier, I mentioned the three types of estrogen produced by the body, estradiol, estrone, and estriol. Researchers have found that estradiol is *probably* safe to use as a treatment; estriol is *definitely* safe; and estrone is *definitely not* safe. Estrone is clearly carcinogenic in excessive amounts, but, as all three are present in the body, it would seem to make sense to supplement with all three in the right balance *if* it is done accurately. A "triple estrogen" is now available that works quite well and is safe when prescribed by a knowledgeable physician.

Unfortunately, very few pharmacists are aware of the availability of triple estrogen. I was recommending estriol to my patients as the only safe estrogen replacement therapy 15 years ago. But the rich were the only ones who could go to England to take advantage of this excellent hormone, so I gave up on it. It was just too frustrating for both the patients and me. Then I heard recently that estriol was now indeed available here. I checked with druggists in three states and they all said it was not listed in their Pharmacopeia as an approved drug.

They were wrong, as there are pharmacies with the knowledge and expertise to compound a safe estrogen product for you. If you have osteoporosis, or a family history of osteoporosis or menopausal symptoms or both, take estriol or the triple estrogen compound. Good sources, if your doctor is unaware of them, are: Women's International Pharmacy, 800-279-5708; Belmar Pharmacy, 800-255-8026; and B&B Pharmacy, 800-231-8905.

There are a couple of ways you can get "endogenous" (i.e., made internally) estrogen and that is by taking boron or DHEA.

Boron

Many of you have been asking where to find a natural form of estrogen. Well, the best answer we've been able to come up with is *boron*. In my special report *What They're Not Telling You About Osteoporosis* I explained that boron is one of the most effective weapons we've seen in the treatment and prevention of osteoporosis.

This little-known mineral fights osteoporosis in two ways. First, it stops the excretion of calcium in the urine — thus maintaining calcium levels in the body. Second, it raises the level of estrogen in postmenopausal women. Studies have shown that the blood levels of estrogen in some women taking boron supplements were as high as the levels found in women undergoing estrogen replacement therapy!

Researchers at the Grand Forks Human Nutrition Research Center in Grand Forks, North Dakota, gave a boron supplement of three mg per day to 12 women ranging in age from 48 to 82. The results were quite remarkable. The boron supplement reduced the loss of calcium in the urine as well as the excretion of magnesium, an unexpected bonus in the treatment of osteoporosis. Within just eight days, the amount of calcium being lost in the urine was reduced by 40 percent, and magnesium loss was cut by 33 percent. And there was even more good news: These postmenopausal women had "markedly elevated" serum estrogen and testosterone levels.

Estrogen and estrogen-like hormones can also be found in some plants, but the amount is usually not high enough to be of any significance. In the few cases where it is high, there is the old problem of absorption. Phytates in plants inhibit the absorption of metals, including boron. You can *ingest* as much as three mg of boron a day by eating plenty of fruit — apples, pears, and grapes. Green vegetables, raw or cooked, and nuts also contain high levels of boron. But *ingesting* and *absorbing* are not the same thing, so it's very important to take a boron supplement.

Boron is toxic, but the lowest reported toxic dose of boron is 45 grams for an adult. The average person gets about 1.5 mg per day; most studies are based on three mg per day. That's 0.000067 of the lowest toxic dose. As with all your vitamins, minerals, and other nutrients, boron should be kept out of the reach of small children. (Although the risk is certainly minimal.)

The fact that boron helps the body conserve calcium, while at the same time raising estrogen levels in older women makes this element a powerful weapon in preventing and reversing osteoporosis — and it may help reduce the severity of your hot flashes.

At the health food store, you'll probably find boron supplements in three and six mg tablets. If you are a small woman, I suggest you buy the three mg size and take one tablet per day. Or you can buy the larger size and take half a tablet each day (this might save you some money). If you are a medium to large woman, purchase the six mg size and take a whole tablet daily.

Cortisone
First Abused and Now Neglected

One of the great medical discoveries of the early 20th century was cortisone. It was miraculous what it would do for arthritis and it was life-saving for Addison's disease, the congenital hypoplasia of the adrenal glands (JFK had it). The rheumatologists rushed to put all their arthritis patients on it; the dermatologists smeared it on everything; and whenever a patient was declared hopeless, he was given the privilege of dying on intravenous cortisone.

Then the unpleasant news began to come in, like one bad weather report after another — bruising, hypertension, diabetes, lowered resistance to infection, cataracts, aggravation of glaucoma, psychoses, acne, peptic ulcer, hirsutism, hypertension, edema, menstrual problems, osteoporosis, sexual dysfunction, moon face, and other signs of Cushing's disease, and balding — whew, no wonder the doctors ran away from cortisone like scalded cats.

In fact, they ran right out of the ball park and many of them never prescribed cortisone again. This is a common occurrence in medicine, where a perfectly fine treatment is completely abandoned because it was misused when introduced on the market with great fanfare.

The problem with cortisone was they were using very large doses without even knowing if the patient was deficient in cortisone. Like testosterone, DHEA, HGH (human growth hormone), thyroid, or any other hormone, if there's not a deficiency, the agent should not be prescribed. You may get dramatic, temporary improvement with large doses of cortisone, but at a terrible price — the disruption of the entire hormonal system.

As I was writing this report, an article appeared in the *London Daily Telegraph* (10/20/96) that illustrates the tragic misunderstandings about cortisone. The headline told the awful story: "Arthritis Drug Eats Into Bones." And what they reported was true. It was a form of cortisone called prednisone and it indeed does cause osteoporosis. The researchers, reporting from the university hospital in Nijmegen, Holland, said, "Prednisone should be limited as much as possible to short-term use until further studies are carried out."

Further studies? There have been zillions of studies documenting the detrimental effects of cortisone used in large doses and using the *wrong type* of cortisone. Such newspaper statements as "Without steroids (cortisone) many people with rheumatoid arthritis would be bedridden" and then following it with: "The use of steroids is increasingly controversial" confuses the public and the doctors as well — is cortisone good or bad?

But now, thanks to the brilliant and painstaking work of Dr. William Jefferies of the University of Virginia School of Medicine, cortisone therapy has been brought into perspective. His work showed that when used properly by a doctor who has done his homework, this powerful compound can do many wonderful things for many suffering people.

After 30 years experience with cortisone, you would think there would be some understanding among clinicians as to how to use it. But most of them *know less* about its use than they did 30 years ago! This is a tragedy for the public because this drug truly is remarkable when used with discretion.

There was nothing wrong with cortisone, we were simply ignorant of how to use the drug. So, with that said, let's look at some of the areas of medicine *crying* for the use of this remarkable substance:

Arthritis: We all remember the sensation that cortisone created when it became widely available in the '60s. People were "cured" practically overnight. But then the terrible after-effects began to appear and many were left more crippled than they would have been without the drug. I had an aunt who was literally destroyed by cortisone and you no doubt know of similar cases.

The secrets in treating arthritis, or any other condition, with cortisone, are:

1. *Determine if the patient has a cortisone deficiency.* You need to get all of your hormones tested with a comprehensive screening. Then take the one you need, if any — and almost everyone over 50 will be short on one or more of the hormones that we now use in practice.

2. Using the proper *minimum dose* that will be effective with the patient. In the days of our youth, we were giving doses *triple* what we should have been giving — and the results you know. Twenty mgs a day is adequate in most arthritis patients.

Acute back pain: There are many treatments for back pain. The reason why is because none of them are dramatically better than the others. Entire specialties are (or were originally) based on the treatment of sore backs — back surgery, chiropractic, and osteopathy. But low doses (i.e. physiologic doses) of hydrocortisone (cortisol) is a treatment that is better than all of them put together. There is, however,

17

no reason not to use manipulative therapy along with cortisol for back pain.

Common cold: Let's leap from the painful to the trivial, relatively speaking, to give you an idea of the versatility of cortisone in medicine. In the past, it has been considered malpractice to give cortisone for a common cold. This was because cortisone had been proven to *mask symptoms of disease* while lowering the body's ability to fight the disease, i.e., causing a depression of the immune system. This was perfectly correct *in the doses that were being given.* But in small *physiologic* doses, as opposed to *pharmacologic* doses, it makes perfect sense to use cortisol for treatment of the common cold *and almost all other diseases.* When a patient is under attack from an acute illness, his body will be deficient in cortisol as the cortisol from the adrenals is being used to fight the invader. With small supplementary doses, there are no adverse effects, only good effects.

So contrary to the common belief among most doctors that cortisone will *decrease* a patient's resistance to infection, when given *in the proper small doses,* the correct cortisone (cortisol) will *increase* the body's defense mechanisms. The proper use of cortisol in small doses can revolutionize the treatment of infections and many other diseases. This adaption to rational cortisone treatment will be slow in coming because of the almost universal ignorance of the proper usage of this hormone.

Acne: One of the most poorly treated conditions in this country is acne. The mainstay of therapy by most doctors, including the dermatologists who should know better, is tetracycline, especially the variant called Minocin (minocycline). *Over 20 years ago* I was railing against the use of this antibiotic in the treatment of acne. It never made sense to me to treat these localized skin infections with antibiotics given by mouth. It's not the way to treat a skin infection and, besides, the condition is basically hormonal and the

18

antibiotics do nothing but temporarily cover up the problem. At the time, I had no idea how bad Minocin really was; it was just the principle of the thing I objected to.

But now, after all these years, Minocin is revealing its ugly side and Wyeth Laboratories is facing millions in damages from kids suffering from liver damage, arthritis, and debilitation, some losing as much as 50 pounds. The doctors ought to get whacked along with Wyeth. In the first place, they shouldn't have given *any* antibiotic for acne. It was lousy medicine to treat a problem that is basically hormonal as though it were a simple skin infection. They should have known better than to believe what some drug salesman told them about how his product is "safer" and "more effective" than the competition. These statements are almost always based on experiments paid for by the company and should be ignored.

The best treatment for acne, although not perfect, is a combination of low-dose cortisol and large doses of vitamin A (100,000 units daily in a divided dose) and 5,000 units of vitamin D daily. If the patient is tested occasionally for liver function, about every three months, this combined therapy can be continued for years with complete safety.

Allergies: Many patients with allergies are found to have an abnormal ACTH test. This is a test to determine if the patient has a faulty pituitary gland that isn't giving the adrenal glands the message to excrete adequate cortisone. Or the patient may have "tired adrenals" and they simply are unable to respond to the stimulus of the ACTH. In either case, these patients will usually respond to small replacement doses of cortisone in the same manner that patients with thyroid deficiency will respond to thyroid and those with a DHEA deficiency will respond to DHEA. These patients, when the deficiency seems to be permanent, can take these small doses of cortisone *indefinitely* with absolutely no untoward effects.

My final thought on this is my major thought on the subject. It is an area that has, as far as I know, been completely overlooked. We have discovered in the past few years that many, in fact most, of our patients over the age of 50, are deficient in one or more of the hormones. Thyroid is, of course, the better known of these. But now we are giving replacement doses of DHEA, testosterone, estrogen, progesterone, and human growth hormone. We now know that the aging process is, to a great degree, due to a deficiency of one or more of these essential hormones. In other words, you are only as young as your hormone status.

Now if this is true of these various hormones, doesn't it stand to reason that the adrenal hormone, cortisol, would be just as important as these other hormones for maintaining health and avoiding premature aging? So my thesis is, and this will cause a fire storm of controversy among defenders of orthodoxy, that many people over the age of 50 need a small, physiologic daily dose of cortisol for the rest of their lives. An under active adrenal cortex is an invitation to disaster because these people do not have the normal defense against disease.

They used to call pneumonia "the old man's friend" because it was what put most of them- away. It killed them because they had exhausted adrenal glands, but pneumonia is a friend I can do without. As you probably know, there are no effective agents for the treatment of viral infections. So when an elderly patient is dying of influenza or viral pneumonia, the doctors stand helplessly by, or do harm by giving antibiotics that further depress the immune system. What these patients need, but seldom get, is physiologic doses of cortisol to help the depleted adrenal glands fight the infection. And many of them, if they were getting the daily small doses of cortisone that we recommend, *wouldn't get the pneumonia in the first place.*

For more information about cortisol, I suggest you read *Safe Uses of Cortisol* by W.M. Jefferies, MD (Charles C. Thomas, Springfield, 111.) or *Resetting the Clock* by Elmer Cranton, MD (M Evans, New York, $21.95).

DHEA and the Story of Duchess

Duchess is right on the cutting edge of biological aging research. After a hysterectomy, she became "fat and fifty" so to speak. She was slowing down, acting matronly and, well, just growing old and portly at a rapid pace. This shouldn't happen to a *dog* — especially a nice dog like Duchess.

Her mistress took her to the University of Wisconsin where they were doing weight-reduction research on dogs. The veterinarian, Dr. Greg MacEwen, put Duchess on DHEA (dehydroepiandrosterone — pronounced D-hi-dro-ep-E-an-dro-stehr-own). The purpose of the treatment with this steroid was to enable Duchess to lose weight, but another remarkable thing happened. She began to act like a puppy with youthful energy and cheerfulness. And the fat melted off — 22 percent of her body weight in two months! And her immune system improved dramatically.

Even more importantly, DHEA appears to be absolutely essential for maintaining the health of humans. The research on the use of DHEA, a hormone from the adrenal glands, has been reported as effective in the treatment of a number of diseases. There is strong evidence that this interesting adrenal compound is essential in the prevention of aging and that it will slow the aging process when the patient has a DHEA deficiency (almost everyone over the age of 50 is deficient). DHEA has the interesting capability of converting into whatever hormone the body needs — it's a "precursor" to most of them. So it's extremely useful for both sexes.

As man ages there is a decrease in the synthesis of protein and thus a decrease in lean body mass and bone mass with an increase in body fat. This fat tends to accumulate around the middle (as you may have noticed), and usually signals the heretofore "inevitable" slide into middle age and beyond. These undesirable body composition changes, as in Duchess, were found by University of California researchers to be accompanied,

21

without exception, by the progressive decline of adrenal secretion of DHEA.

The importance of DHEA deficiency in human aging, and its importance in many other diseases, is puzzling because no mammalians, except man and monkeys, have the ability to synthesize and secrete DHEA. In fact, the adrenals of humans and primates manufacture more DHEA than all the other hormones combined, so it is the most abundant hormone in the bloodstream. It makes sense that the production of DHEA would be prodigious, as it converts into the other hormones as needed, but why don't other animal species do the same thing? It seems the Creator gave us a backup system that He denied to most of the species. It is interesting to note that when animals, like Duchess, are given DHEA, they respond in a positive way, just as humans do.

Research over the past 10 years, reported in the *New England Journal of Medicine* and other respected journals, has shown that a low DHEA level in the blood is associated with increased heart disease, breast cancer, and a decline in the competence of the immune system. In fact, the correlation of DHEA levels with heart attacks and breast cancer is so strong that all doctors should be checking the DHEA level on all patients over 50. As you know from reading my columns over the years, serum cholesterol is *not* an accurate predictor of heart disease. Serum DHEA levels should replace it for predictive purposes, but most doctors don't even know what DHEA is!

As for its importance in predicting breast cancer, in a long-term study of 5,000 women it was found that DHEA levels fell drastically *up to nine years* before the onset of clinically proven breast cancer. The researchers concluded that *the highest risk factor for breast cancer was a low level of DHEA.*

Dr. Eric Braverman, the director of Path Medical/Path Foundation in Princeton, New Jersey, had this to say about DHEA and the treatment of cancer in *DHEA, A Practical*

Guide: "We have found DHEA, although not a magic bullet or panacea, to be useful in a variety of conditions such as chronic fatigue, burns, Reiter's syndrome, idiopathic thrombocytopenic purpura, menopause, immune deficiencies, memory problems, and even certain forms of cancer. We've given high doses of DHEA, up to 1,000 mg a day, to some terminal cancer cases, such as pancreatic cancer, and noticed that it was of benefit. Other anecdotal cases include shrinkage of lymphomas. We are experimenting using DHEA in combination with chemotherapy or other modalities." (Avery, 1996) [Stick with the "other modalities," Doc.]

Research at the University of California revealed that for every microgram per cc increase in blood levels of DHEA, *death by all causes was diminished by 36 percent.* In men 50 to 70, there was a *48 percent decrease in death from heart attacks.* Another study, reported in the *New England Journal of Medicine,* of 242 men between the ages of 50 and 79 concluded: "Those individuals with higher DHEA-S [DHEA sulfate] levels lived longer and had a much lower risk of heart disease."

There is also evidence that DHEA will work in the treatment of diabetes. Dr. Alan Gaby writes in *Holistic Medicine* (Spring 1993), "A certain inbred strain of mice has a genetic disorder which causes them to develop diabetes. Their pancreatic beta-cells, those cells in the pancreas which make insulin, are also spontaneously destroyed during the course of their lifetime. When this strain of mice was given 0.4 percent DHEA in their diet, the diabetes was rapidly reversed and the beta-cells were preserved. In a study of other animals without this genetic disorder. DHEA reduced the severity of diabetes resulting from administering a diabetes-inducing chemical called streptozotocin."

In another study, researchers at the University of California, La Jolla, studied the effects of DHEA on 13 men and 17 women for six months. They were given a small dose (50 mg) of DHEA daily and then the results were compared with a placebo group that received only dummy capsules. Blood levels of the hormone were quickly restored to those of a 20-year-old. The positive findings in the treated group were impressive whereas the patients in the placebo group showed no significant positive changes.

The majority of the patients on DHEA reported increased energy, deeper sleep, improved mood, a more relaxed feeling and a better ability to handle stressful events. The decrease in "middle-age spread" was quite discernible in most patients, but not in the placebo group.

DHEA deficiency is clearly associated with memory loss as medical school studies have shown that mental-function test scores improve and patients consistently report an improvement in memory after taking DHEA.

There is bogus DHEA in the health food stores. These are herbal preparations that have no hormone effect and so they should be avoided. If you do not believe this, you can check it yourself by taking the recommended herb for a few weeks and then having your DHEA sulfate level checked and compared with the one you had taken before starting the "DHEA-containing" herbal.

Legitimate DHEA is also available in health food stores in pharmacologically adequate doses, but be sure you are getting the real thing. This hormone is too important to your health to not make sure you are getting the potency you need. If you're in doubt, the lab that produces Healthy Resolve's DHEA has guaranteed its potency. Make sure your brand has a similar guarantee.

I strongly recommend that if you are over 50, get a blood test for your DHEA-S level. If your level is below that of a normal 30-year-old, I recommend that you take DHEA. You will not have to go to a doctor to get it, but I don't think it is wise to take a hormone, even a safe one like DHEA, without checking your blood level to see if you really need it.

The following is a list of illnesses that can benefit from taking DHEA:

Post menopausal relief	Antiobesity
Improved athletic performance	Antiviral
Lupus erythematosus	Antidiabetic
Immune system stimulant	Anticancer
Thymus gland protector	Antidepressant
Alzheimer's disease	Antidementia
Improved memory	Heart protector
Improved learning	Improved sleep
Antiatherosclerotic	Anti-aging effect
Decrease in joint pain	Increased muscle mass
Chronic fatigue syndrome	

That's a lot of claims. While I don't think DHEA is going to work in all these conditions all the time, I think it's important for general health in most people over 50. It may also be beneficial for some even younger, as the DHEA level starts falling after age 30.

A note on Alzheimer's disease and DHEA: Brain tissue, under normal conditions, contains 6.5 times more DHEA than the circulating blood. Alzheimer's sufferers have low blood levels of DHEA — 48 percent less than normal. Which is cause and which is effect? That is, does Alzheimer's disease depress DHEA levels or does a low DHEA contribute to the disease? It's the old question: "Which came first, the chicken or the egg?" With DHEA and Alzheimer's, we simply don't know, yet. Obviously, it's a good idea to take DHEA is you're deficient.

DHEA will not enable you to live forever, but it may cause a dramatic increase in your longevity, if you do the other things right. I should know. I'm a regular user of DHEA and it does wonders for me. I usually take around 200 mg, but most people don't need more than 50-100 mg.

New research is finding that you should take DHEA in the morning before breakfast or sublingually (letting it dissolve under your tongue). DHEA isn't fat-soluble so if you have any fat in your dinner, such as olive oil in your salad or some nice lamb chops with the fat on them, it will block the absorption of the DHEA. This problem can be alleviated by taking the tablet sublingually. This will bypass the intestinal tract and you can take it anytime you like. This is the best way to take DHEA, and Healthy Resolve has made its DHEA to dissolve very efficiently this way. I have to admit that it doesn't taste very good, though. If you can handle the taste, do it sublingually. Otherwise, take it with water an hour before breakfast.

Talk to a doctor who understands DHEA and see what he recommends for you. (We will have information on how to find a doctor at the end of this report.)

Ref: *Journal of Clinical Endocrinology and Metabolism,* 1994, Vol. 78, No. 6; Personal communication with Elmer Cranton, M.D.; *Journal of Neuroscience Research,* 1987, 17(3) pp 225-34; *Chicago Tribune,* December 9, 1991.

Pregnenolone

Another "multiple-action," precursor hormone like DHEA is pregnenolone. It combines with cholesterol to make another hormone, which goes on to produce DHEA. So do you need both? We don't know for sure. But if you take pregnenolone (It won't make you pregnant, although the name might make you wonder) instead of DHEA, it will produce DHEA as well as progesterone and other hormones from the adrenal and sex glands.

I think both should be taken, as pregnenolone seems to have some unique health-enhancing properties of its own. It seems to have, in experimental animals at least, powerful memory-enhancing qualities. It is free of serious side effects and is effective in doses smaller than those needed for therapeutic effect with DHEA. With DHEA, the effective dose ranges from 25 to 500 mgs, but pregnenolone requires only a dose of 5 to 100 mgs. Pregnenolone, DHEA, and natural progesterone are all extracted from wild yams. Pregnenolone is available without a prescription from Women's International Pharmacy, mentioned above, and from Scientific Consulting Service, 800-333-7414.

But, as with DHEA, I don't think you should take these hormones without the supervision of a doctor. He will be able to give you the right dosage for your condition.

Natural Progesterone

I started using natural progesterone for the treatment of premenstrual syndrome (PMS) in 1982. I had gone to England to study with Dr. Katherina Dalton, the originator of this excellent therapy for a vexing problem. I ran into a buzz saw of emotion in Atlanta, Georgia, where I had only been practicing for a year. Having escaped the wrath of the Florida medical priesthood, the last thing I wanted at this juncture in my career was more controversy. In medicine, innovation is a sure road to insolvency and I had seen enough of that. I was definitely ready for some solvency — but it was not to be.

A reporter for the *Atlanta Journal* called and interviewed me for the better part of an hour. Unknown to me, she had already interviewed a professor of gynecology at Emory University who told her that "Douglass is full of crap." So her mind was made up when she called me. She then wrote a blistering editorial about my flaming quackery and male chauvinism.

Following this devastating attack by the *Journal*, I received anonymous threatening phone calls and a letter

27

from a local company deploring my very existence in our wonderful town with the greatest medical facilities in the world, etc., etc. It was signed by 20 of their employees, male and female!

But I was finally vindicated eight years later. I was preparing to move to Russia when I saw an interview on TV concerning the treatment of PMS. The learned professor from Emory (a different one) said: "Yes, this is a serious situation in many women. We now have an effective therapy using a natural progesterone. PMS is basically a progesterone deficiency." I felt a little satisfaction from this, but not enough to make up for the insults and the harm to my practice.

The source of natural progesterone is from plants, particularly wild yams and soy beans. When taken in pill form, or rubbed on the skin (transdermal application), the plant saponins are converted to a type of natural progesterone that is identical in structure to the progesterone produced by the body.

The reports I've seen show some remarkable success with the transdermal application of a cream containing wild yam.

A 1990 study involving 63 post menopausal women with osteoporosis showed that those using the transdermal cream had a more than seven percent *increase* in bone mass during the study's first year, and more than five percent increase during the second.

Those results are impressive. If you can find this transdermal cream (I've seen it occasionally in more sophisticated health food stores), rub your hands and arms with it twice a day. If it is not available in your area, try taking the wild yam herb itself. This is commonly available in pill form (two, twice a day).

Natural progesterone is also available by capsule or rectal solution and is more effective than the creams, especially for menopause and premenstrual syndrome. You must go to a qualified medical doctor for this, as it is a prescription item.

A Hormone You Didn't Know
You Were Taking — Calciferol

Millions of American women flock to GNC for their anti-osteoporosis calcium pills without benefit of the full story — *the necessity of vitamin D in adequate doses.*

Vitamin D, is the key to calcium supplementation: You can take all the calcium pills you want, but if your body isn't assimilating the calcium (isn't using it), the calcium can't do the job.

Most people are surprised to hear that vitamin D (calciferol) is a hormone. Somehow, sunshine manufactures vitamin D in the skin. We know this because a few hours in the sun increases the vitamin D levels in the blood. But it's not so easy once you're passed middle age. Studies have shown that women in their 60s can't manufacture vitamin D from sunshine — at least they can't do it efficiently any more. That's why it's important for older women to supplement their diet with vitamin D capsules. Once you're in your 60's, it's essential.

They taught us in medical school that vitamin D was highly toxic and that, although some calciferol in the diet was essential, an excess could have dire consequences, the worst consequence being hardening of the arteries. This is absolutely incorrect and very high doses of vitamin D are completely safe. Because of this phobia about calciferol, the same "medical phobia" we had to fight concerning vitamin C and vitamin A, millions of people have been denied maximum health due to calcium deficiency secondary to the lack of the Vitamin D hormone in their diet. And now it is being exacerbated by patients being told by their doctor to stay out of the sun!

The question of toxicity of vitamin D should have been laid to rest by the report from the University of Chicago, College of Medicine, which revealed the astounding facts on vitamin D "toxicity." Their studies on hundreds of humans

29

and 64 dogs revealed that it's one of the *least* toxic of the "vitamins." A 200-pound man can take *two million* units of vitamin D per day with absolutely no adverse effects. The government's "recommended daily allowance" for this vital nutrient is a paltry 400 units — 0.04 percent of the safe two-m'AYion unit dose. (Your body can manufacture 10,000 units on a sunny day at the beach, if you are young and healthy.)

The Chicago researchers did find toxicity at 25 *million* units per day, but Dr. C. Reynolds, of Louisiana State University, said that the toxic effect was probably due to impurities in the earlier batches of the vitamins, as the Chicago report was published in 1937!

But today, about 60 years later, doctors, and your omniscient government, still think the vitamin D hormone is a dangerous substance. In the case of the government, the answer for this blindness is simple stupidity. As for the doctors, there are two reasons for their scientific myopia: a slavish dependence on government data and a lack of interest in the nutritional literature.

There is no better example of medical hypocrisy than the case of Carl J. Reich, M.D., and his fight for common sense in the use of calcium and vitamin D in osteoporosis and other deficiency diseases.

Soon after he graduated from medical school, Dr. Reich determined from an intensive reading of the scientific literature that there was a high probability that many chronic diseases, from arthritis to osteoporosis, were due to a calcium deficiency. This deficiency was due, he reasoned, to lack of assimilation of the calcium due to a vitamin D deficiency. He knew what you now know: There can be *no* absorption of calcium without the presence of vitamin D in the small intestine.

Over a 30-year period, Dr. Reich treated many thousands of patients with a combination of vitamin D, calcium, and magnesium and had phenomenal results. Even asthma, rheumatoid, and osteoarthritis patients improved dramatically in 60-90 percent of the cases. Reich had such excellent results, with a huge practice and thousands of grateful patients singing his praises, that the medical "oracles" could no longer tolerate this threat to their religious temple, so they revoked his license to practice. Although he had never had a complaint from a patient, the medical soviet decided that he was a "potential danger." (Danger to whom they did not say.)

What Dr. Reich did was simple and it is what you should do to prevent osteoporosis or ameliorate it if you are already afflicted with it. (Your asthma or arthritis may also improve.)

Reich recognized the importance of the body's acidity in the etiology of disease and that proper assimilation of minerals, like calcium, could not take place without the body being on the alkaline side.

He devised a simple test using a test tape obtainable from any drug store. Do the test between meals. Generate some saliva a few times and spit it out. Then, with some fresh saliva in your mouth, lick it onto the tape. The healthiest range is dark blue (Ph of 7.5) to medium blue (Ph of 7:0). If the tape shows a blue-green or yellow, your fluids are in the acidic range and you are calcium deficient. (The test tapes are called Hydrion Papers and they are made by Micro Essential Laboratory, Brooklyn, N.Y. 11210 or plain Nitrazine strips available at the drug store will do.)

Urine can be tested rather than saliva. If the urine Ph is 7.0 or higher, vitamin D supplementation is not necessary.

If you are an adult of normal size, you should immediately begin taking 50,000 units of vitamin A daily (check with your doctor before taking this much A), 5,000 units of vitamin D, and 1,000 mgs of calcium. When the saliva test results improve, cut back to 2,500 units of D and continue the 50,000 units of vitamin A, and the 1,000 mg of calcium. Continue to check your saliva or urine weekly.

31

Dr. Reich will probably never be honored for his significant contribution to the health of mankind, but he would be pleased to know that his gift to us all has gone far beyond his practice.

A researcher in Holland has also rediscovered vitamin D. Dr. Gees Vermeer of the University of Maastricht found that women who lose abnormally high amounts of calcium through their urine could *cut the loss by up to 50 percent* by taking adequate amounts of vitamin D. But "adequate amounts" mean different things to different people.

Dr. Hector F. DeLuca, a biochemist at the University of Wisconsin, has taken vitamin D to a new level of respect. "Just like vitamin C isn't just for breakfast anymore, so vitamin D isn't just for bones anymore," he said. Vitamin D has proven to have a wealth of effects in tissues other than bones. It acts like a potent steroid hormone igniting wide-scale gene activity in skin, pancreas, parathyroid, breast, and ovaries. It has been found to be possibly effective in the treatment of colon and breast cancer. In cell studies, calciferol has been found to show a suppression, of the growth of cancer cells and a change to more normal cells.

The skin not only serves as a manufacturing facility for vitamin D, but it turns out to be an organ that must have vitamin D as a nutrient. It has been found effective in the treatment of psoriasis and contact dermatitis (an inflammation of the skin from allergy or chemical sensitivity) when given by mouth and is even effective by cream in cases of psoriasis.

I discussed the toxicity issue with Dr. DeLuca, who is possibly *the* foremost expert in the world on vitamin D. He said that 5,000 units is very safe in a normal person and that 10,000 units was probably safe. He didn't say he recommended that you take that much; he just said it was safe if there was no kidney or liver compromise. I don't want to misquote him.

I wasn't able to verify the 1937 University of Chicago research. It's difficult to trace research that is 60 years old.

You don't need to take a million units of vitamin D anyway — 5,000-10,000 units will do.

As your betters in the PDA think vitamin D is toxic, you can't get it in conveniently large doses as you can vitamin A. The largest dose is 400 international units. If you don't mind doing a lot of swallowing, I recommend that you take at least 10 capsules a day. *That is not a large dose,* but if you are skeptical, have your doctor check your liver and kidney function every three months. Not one doctor in a hundred understands the importance or the biology of vitamin D. So you must decide whether you want to debate the issue with him about the liver and kidney test or just tell him you have hepatophobia.

A number of studies have shown that calciferol promotes hardening of the arteries, atherosclerosis, in experimental animals, possibly from folic acid inhibition. Animal studies don't always correlate with human physiology and the doses required to have this effect in animals is higher than what we recommend. But to be on the safe side, take 1,600 micrograms of folic acid along with your 5,000 units of vitamin D daily.

Testosterone for Men and Women

For many of you, the very mention of testosterone brings visions of large, greedy athletes who have artificially increased their muscle mass by taking anabolic steroids (testosterone). Or perhaps you see images of some sex-crazed maniac who can very easily become aggressive, even violent. Unfortunately, these images are often justified. It wasn't too long ago that Lyle Alzado, the All-Pro defensive lineman for the Los Angeles Raiders, went on a crusade exposing the terrible side effects of large amounts of steroids. He later died from a brain tumor caused by *heavy* steroid use.

It's these very stigmas that have caused doctors to shy away from using testosterone for aging males. They have seen how improper use can cause cancer, high blood pressure, or hardening of the arteries. And they weren't about to use it on women as it would cause virilism, acne, an increase in libido (true), baldness, and other terrible things. Now we know that all of the problems caused by this hormone were usually due to overdose, uninformed doctors, and improper use.

The good news is that testosterone *is* a beneficial hormone if used correctly. Ample research now indicates that testosterone is our most neglected hormone and when it's properly used is a marvelous adjunct in the fight against aging — in both sexes. And it does more than just fight aging.

One of my colleagues, Dr. Richard S. Wilkinson, related the following case at a medical meeting in Virginia Beach last year.

One of his patients, a wealthy research physicist, began "going down hill" at the age of 49. He started suffering from allergies and had a ruptured disc in his back. At age 55, a severe heart irregularity was added to his growing list of complaints. In desperation he finally went to the world-famous Scripts Clinic in southern California. After an extensive and expensive workup, they found nothing, but the doctors gave him the hardly encouraging news that he was "aging a little faster than normal — that's life and that's the hand that was dealt to you."

This "extensive and expensive" workup did not include a check on his blood testosterone levels. As so often happens with men in the other fields of science when they go to a doctor, the patient became disillusioned and sought his own answers. As a physicist, he was knowledgeable in the field of feedback mechanisms and concluded that his problem must be related to hormones, which are one of the body's main feedback control systems.

After visiting various experts, including a professor of endocrinology at the UCLA Medical School, he found a wholistically oriented doctor who understood what he was trying to do and worked with him to regulate his body's hormones. His new doctor was able to home in on the problem quickly, as he knew what tests the Scripts experts seldom or never do - a test of the thyroid with underarm temperatures and a blood testosterone test. The doctor scored a thousand on both tests: The patient had both low thyroid function and a low blood testosterone level.

Immediately, the doctor began proper treatment and the brilliant physicist was virtually rejuvenated and probably saved from an early death.

As you can see, some practitioners are finally starting to realize that the function of the testicles should be taken seriously in health related matters — not just sexual matters. But it's taken 145 years. Back in 1849, the science of endocrinology was born through the work of German physiologist Arnold Berthold. Professor Berthold performed a simple experiment that proved beyond a doubt that something in the testicles made a rooster a rooster — and a man a man.

Berthold removed the testicles from four roosters, thus making them capons. He then gave testicles back to two of the four birds by implanting a testicle into their abdominal walls. The "emasculated," as we now call it, roosters remained fat and lazy capons with no interest in fighting or copulating. The cocks that were rewarded with testicles strutted, crowed, fought ferociously, and continually chased the ladies — nothing ambiguous about *that* experiment.

In spite of Berthold's experiments and many present-day success stories, modern medicine has held tightly to the age-old myths that testosterone therapy is dangerous and could, in fact, increase the likelihood of a heart attack, cancer, or some other dastardly disease.

But now we've found that the exact *opposite* is true. Men who have had heart attacks tend to have *low* testosterone levels. Professor Gerald B. Phillips, M.D., of Columbia University Medical School studied 55 men undergoing X-ray exams of their arteries and found that those with a lower testosterone level had higher degrees of heart disease, i.e., blockage of the coronary arteries. He also found that the protective HDL cholesterol levels were higher in men with higher testosterone levels.

Consistent with the above report, Dr. Maurice A. Lesser studied the effect of testosterone in 100 cases of angina pectoris, which is caused by either spasm or blockage of the arteries in the heart. Testosterone injections had a remarkable result: Out of the 100 cases, 91 showed "moderate to marked" improvement in their chest pain. Only nine had no improvement at all. In the cases showing improvement, both the frequency and the severity of the attacks were reduced.

The evidence for serious toxicity or permanent adverse effects from the proper use of testosterone simply is not there. In fact, testosterone has been proven to be *protective* against cancer, in women as well as in men. It has been suggested that testosterone is contraindicated in men with cancer of the prostate. In view of the hormone's protective effect in other cancers, I doubt the validity of this supposition.

Another surprising action of testosterone is its anticoagulant effect. It may prove to be far safer than aspirin or Coumadin and, while keeping the blood "thin," it bestows the other benefits depicted in this report.

Testosterone also has an interesting effect on the rhythm of the heart. You saw in the story of the physicist how his heart irregularity was cleared completely with testosterone therapy. This cardiac effect was confirmed in a study reported in the *British Heart Journal* in which it was found that the "male hormone" had a significant effect on a heart with a depressed electrical system.

Even more significant is the research done in Japan on the prevention of stroke with testosterone therapy. The Japanese claim to have significantly reduced the incidence and the severity of stroke with testosterone injections.

Michael Hansen, M.D., claims that 20 percent of patients with "stroke-like" symptoms, i.e., a temporary paralysis or numbness called transient ischemic attack, or TIA, will have a stroke within two years "if there is no intervention." By "intervention" he means testosterone therapy. With testosterone the incidence of stroke plummets from 20 percent to two percent.

Another remarkable effect of testosterone is in the control of blood sugar. Even with severe diabetes, testosterone therapy can be of great benefit including treatment of the dreaded diabetic retinopathy, which leads to blindness. Dr. M.L. Tainter reported in the *New York State Journal of Medicine* that vision was improved, or at least stopped deteriorating, in 75 percent of cases treated with testosterone.

While it may sound like testosterone is a wonder drug that will cure everything and keep you living forever, it's not. But it is truly amazing what is sometimes possible by treating with this neglected hormone.

But in order to put testosterone in proper perspective, we need to stop thinking of it in terms of sex. While this is obviously one of its important roles, there is much more to this remarkable hormone than that. *Testosterone is a metabolic powerhouse* of amazing versatility. It is one of the major regulators of sugar, fat, and protein metabolism. In other words, testosterone is one of the keys, and perhaps the most important key, to good health and a long life.

And when I say "long life," I am not engaging in idle speculation. Impotence is a definite alarm bell in males. When you become impotent, you can count on dying about 20 years later. As your sexual ability deteriorates, everything else deteriorates in tandem.

Actually, men start dying after the age of 25 as there is a gradual and steady decline of free blood testosterone. (There may be a lot of testosterone bound up with protein, but it is about as useful as water surrounded by marble.) At age 25, the average free testosterone level is about 200 pg/ml. (Don't worry about what the units mean.) At age 80, free testosterone is about 10 pg/ml.

Let's look at the incidence of impotence in our culture and see where you or your spouse fits:

Age	Rate of impotence
40	2 percent of men are impotent
50	5 percent
60	18 percent
70	27 percent
80	75 percent

As you can see, there *is* a menopause in men and it's called the andropause. It is not as dramatic in onset as the menopause in women, but it is a reality — and devastating in its effects. The andropausal man will experience specific disease conditions as well as general symptoms that make life a burden. These symptoms include weakness, impotence, pain, stiffness, drooping muscles, depression, irritability, and excessive sweating with intolerance to heat, just to mention the general stuff. It gets worse from there. Most women do not hesitate to complain to the doctor about their "change of life," but most men suffer in silence and accept it as the inevitability of aging. Unfortunately, so do most doctors.

But, as with the case of the research physicist we mentioned earlier, *many of these problems will completely disappear with proper testosterone therapy.*

If that promise sounds too good to be true, let me assure you, it isn't. And the story gets better!

With all the exciting new research on testosterone, I think the biggest surprise is the discovery of how absolutely vital the hormone is for females. While "anabolic therapy," as it is called, has been grossly neglected in males, it is essentially unheard of in the treatment of females. That's why this report is *must* reading for both sexes.

Although a female only needs 10 percent of the testosterone level men need for maximum health, they need this 10 percent just as much as men need their proper quota. Many postmenopausal women have essentially *no* testosterone. So they have *two* major problems: menopause *and* andropause. Now, that's just not fair!

Testosterone is effective in the treatment and prevention of bone loss. That means it's a natural for treating osteoporosis. For many years, estrogen has been used to treat osteoporosis, but the results have been inconclusive. I think it's a waste of time and money, to say nothing of the cancer risk. Testosterone therapy is clearly more effective than estrogen and safer (completely safe, in fact).

Many of you know that I have decried the indiscriminate use of synthetic estrogen and synthetic progesterone (the two female hormones) for years, because there is strong evidence that they are carcinogenic, especially concerning cancer of the breast. In regard to the use of synthetic testosterone, let me remind you that I have not abandoned all of conventional medicine and I have not accepted uncritically all of alternative medicine — there is some good and bad to be found in both.

It is true that there is an increase in the incidence of breast cancer in women taking synthetic estrogen (Premarin). But natural estrogen seems to be unrelated to breast cancer as there is an *increase* in this disease after menopause, when estrogen decreases. Put another way, a woman's intrinsic estrogen (and progesterone, the other female hormone) seem to be protective and the synthetics, cancer-promoting. But the testosterone factor, usually ignored in this equation, may be far more important than both of the female hormones put together.

After menopause, there is a dramatic decrease in androgens (testosterone). These androgens are protective against breast cancer and are probably the key to prevention. It has been assumed that the changes seen after menopause in women — the deepening voice, the increase in hair, an increase in libido — are due to a relative increase in testosterone. But the opposite seems to be true. This is a little confusing, because testosterone definitely drops off at menopause; it doesn't increase. Have we been missing the boat here? We know that progesterone, the other female hormone, is protective against breast cancer. But testosterone is 1,000 times more protective than progesterone.

It seems to me that we need to stop thinking of estrogen, progesterone, and testosterone as "male" or "female" hormones, because they are probably equally important, in the right proportion, in both sexes. It's certainly true in women and so it follows, at least to me, that the same will prove to be true in men. As Dr. Wilkinson's physicist patient found out on his own, *balance* is the key.

C.W. Lovell, M.D., of the Baton Rouge Menopause Clinic, has confirmed the importance of hormonal balance in the prevention of breast cancer. In the treatment of 4,000 patients, in which he used a combination of estrogen (estradiol) and testosterone, he has reduced the incidence of breast cancer to *less than half* the national average. Using another statistic, his results are even more impressive. On average, there is one cancer discovered for every 100 mammograms performed. In those patients on testosterone therapy, there is only one cancer in every 1,000 mammograms — a decrease of 90 percent!

With testosterone therapy, there is a medical sea change in the offing for the treatment of andropause, menopause, aging, diabetes, cardiovascular disease, osteoporosis, and cancer.

If you wait for conventional medicine to accept and employ this remarkable therapy, you may be in heaven looking down and saying: "I *told* you I needed my hormones balanced."

If you decide to take testosterone therapy, there are a couple of things you need to know. First, your mate should consider taking the therapy, too. Otherwise there may be some serious conflicts in your sex life leading to some problems you can do without. *Partners* have to be in balance, too! Second, make sure that your doctor *does not* use methyl-testosterone for the treatment. The United States is the only country that still uses this particular synthetic hormone and there's a reason for that. It is very well documented that methyl-testosterone is harmful to the liver. Doctors in Europe won't touch the stuff.

Ref: *Arteriosclerosis and Thrombosis*, 14:701-706, 1994; *Journal of Clinical Endocrinology*, 1946:6;549-557; *Lancet, July 21,1962: US-132; British Journal of Haematology*, 1972,22,543; *British Heart Journal*, 1977,39,1217-1222; *Japanese Circulation Journal*, 39, March 1975, 285ff; *New York State Journal of Medicine*, April 15, 1964, lOOlff; *Royal College of General Practitioners Members' Reference Handbook*, 1994; *Journal of Clinical Endocrinology and Metabolism*, June 1994; *Journal of Clinical Endocrinology and Metabolism*, November 1994; *Harvard Health Letter*, July 1994.

A Hormone Approved for Osteoporosis Can Also Treat Pain

We have told you about DHEA, from the adrenal glands, testosterone, progesterone, and now the story on another remarkable hormone that is manufactured by the "C cells" in the thyroid gland. It's called *calcitonin*.

What's so remarkable about calcitonin? This hormone stops the escape of bone in osteoporosis, a process called "resorption," by suppressing the cells that "eat" bone, called osteoclasts. Research has shown beyond a doubt that

41

calcitonin counteracts both early and well-established osteo-porosis. Unfortunately, the levels of this hormone are much lower in women, which has a direct bearing on osteoporosis in elderly women.

Equally remarkable, calcitonin relieves the terrible and disabling pain of compression fractures of the spine. The method of action in this pain relief is not understood, but calcitonin seems to have an independent pain-relieving activity, probably mediated in the brain. One study of patients with "phantom-limb syndrome" (an amputee, for instance, will experience severe pain in a "foot" that is no longer there) found that 80 percent of them experienced great relief that lasted from many hours to a week with calcitonin therapy. One even went three months without pain.

Diabetic neuropathy, the nerve pain in the extremities experienced by diabetics, is also dramatically relieved in a large percentage of patients treated with calcitonin.

As stated above, it is a mystery as to how calcitonin re-lieves pain in such disparate diseases as diabetic neuropathy and phantom-limb. There are all s.orts of scientific explana-tions, such as "boosting of beta-endorphin levels," but no one really knows for sure. There is no doubt, though, that it's an excellent pain reliever with no apparent addictive properties.

The drug is now considered so important, and is so safe, that experts are suggesting it be used in a wide variety of neurological diseases and bone diseases not responding to other treatments. This includes ataxia (lack of muscular coordination), spastic conditions, paralysis of the legs (paraplegia), paralysis of the cranial nerves (the major nerves that come from the brain and upper neck), bone pain, neurologic complications following injuries, osteoporosis, and just about any other condition you can think of related to nerves and bones, including even doses of calcitonin before and after routine orthopedic surgery.

The problem in the United States, as you can readily guess, has been that the PDA would not allow the sale of calcitonin, until recently. The literature is extensive on the benefits of this hormone and it has been used in Europe for many years with complete safety. The motto in this country has become: "If you want the latest in effective and safe treatment for your disease, call your travel agent.[55] We still have good airlines here.

Finally, calcitonin has been released in an injectable form, and a nasal spray has also been "approved[55] by your doctors[5] bosses at the PDA. The spray has been found to be very effective in an array of conditions, such as pain from bone fractures that is often so severe it causes complete disability, and for the treatment of osteoporosis. Some researchers believe that the nasal spray is as effective as the injection form.

The downside to this wonderful advance in hormone therapy is that it is derived from salmon and may cause an allergic reaction in some patients. The synthetic injection form used in Europe seems to be essentially free of side effects.

Keep in mind that the big brothers at the PDA have only approved calcitonin nasal spray (Miacalcin, Sandoz Co.) and the injectable for the prevention of osteoporosis. But once the cat is out of the bag, the PDA admits that doctors are not breaking the law by using the hormone for other diseases in which they think there may be a benefit.

Action to take: If you have any of the conditions mentioned above, and you are not getting relief, or the condition is getting worse, ask your doctor about calcitonin therapy. If the nasal spray doesn't work, I wouldn't give up. Go to Europe and consult with a neurologist or orthopedist familiar with the drug. You can get a list of forward-thinking European doctors, and in other parts of the world as well, from ACAM (23121 Verdugo Drive, Suite 204, Laguna Hills, CA 92653, 800-532-3688 or 714-583-7666) and IOMA (P.O. Box 891954, Oklahoma City, OK 73189, 405-634-7320).

Ref: *Pain,* 1992,48:21-27; *Lancet,* 1992,339:746-747; 1990, 336:449; *American Journal of Medicine,* 1974,56:858-866; Arthritis and Rheumatism, 1980,23:1139-1147; *New England Journal of Medicine,* 1981,304:269-278; *Chronic Pain Letter,* Vol. XII, #5, 1995.

The Miraculous Calming
Effects of Melatonin

Insomnia has become such a major problem for many elderly Americans that sleeping pills are now a multimillion dollar business. And while the medical profession has been asleep, the great unlettered population has tried valiantly (but largely unsuccessfully) to solve this "Insomnia of the Aged" problem. "Sleep clinics" around the U.S. have been raking it in with expensive testing procedures, biofeedback, acupuncture, hypnosis, psychological counseling, and many useless soporifics.

But now melatonin, a natural sleep inducer, is putting these clinics out of business. It's popularity has grown so rapidly that in the last few monthsj I've received a mound of mail and countless phone calls asking me what I think of this "miracle hormone."

The truth about melatonin is that it truly could prove to be a miracle hormone. It acts as an aphrodisiac, sex organ rejuvenator, promoter of zinc absorption (*very* important for males), thyroid stimulator, soporific, anti-stress agent, cancer fighter, and even a contraceptive!

The relationship between cancer and melatonin is quite exciting both from the standpoint of prevention and treatment. Blind women the world over have a high level of circulating melatonin and a low risk of developing breast cancer. Studies with rats have proven that melatonin will dramatically reduce the rate of growth of prostate cancer in these experimental animals.

Another study from Britain gives us encouraging news in the treatment of cancer with this remarkable compound. The researchers, reporting in the June 1993, *British Journal of Cancer,* found a remarkable response in *advanced cancers* to melatonin therapy. There was a positive response of 23 percent. That may not sound very impressive, but remember, these were far-advanced, *terminal* cases. So the results were impressive indeed.

Some of you have asked about the new best-seller, *The Melatonin Miracle.* It's a good book, but I think it promises too much in that it implies that melatonin will cure just about everything. You know the old saying: "If it claims to cure everything, then it probably cures nothing." But in this case, it does have a broad spectrum action due to its influence on other glands in the body. It works directly on the pituitary and thus affects all the endocrine glands. It has a direct control over the thymus gland, which is vital to your immune system. The pineal contains epithalamin, which is probably just as important as melatonin, but we know little about it, and vasopressin, which is involved in milk production and prolactin, also connected to milk production.

But nothing is perfect, including melatonin. Some unfortunate people are *stimulated* by melatonin. Others experience nightmares. And there are a few contraindications: Patients on cortisone should not take melatonin, as melatonin will counteract the action of the cortisone. With some illnesses controlled by cortisone, this could be serious. Severe mental illness might be made worse by melatonin and allergies may also be exacerbated.

It follows that melatonin should be used with caution when other drugs are being taken, especially other soporific agents, such as Valium. There is no place for melatonin, or any other hormone, in the treatment of healthy children. And pregnant women should avoid all sedatives, both natural and synthetic.

As I mentioned earlier in this report, the pharmaceutical industry is working furiously to panic Congress to restrict melatonin to doctors' prescriptions. With this restriction, the "ethical" drug pushers can increase the price 5-10 times because of an artificially restricted market. And, of course, the doctors will be able to charge a fee for writing the prescription.

The head commando in this drive to deny the people easy access to this hormone is Dr. Richard Wurtman, who is carrying out his war under the aegis of the Massachusetts Institute of Technology (MIT). He sends out a stern form letter on MIT stationary to desperate insomniacs warning against using melatonin until it becomes a regulated drug.

What Dr. Wurtman *doesn't* mention in his attempt to stop the sales of melatonin in health food stores is that *he owns a million shares of Interneuron Corp. worth $6 million.* The company has obtained the rights to a patent application for the use of melatonin as a soporific agent. Never trust a researcher, no matter what letterhead he uses, until you check his stock portfolio.

Action to Take

1. There is no doubt about it; melatonin is a "miracle hormone" if there ever was one and I am certain there will be other miracles coming forth from the little pineal power house. Start taking melatonin right away — don't wait for "further studies."

Most melatonin supplements come in three mg tablets. But if you're in your early 40s, that's three times as much as you need (one mg). If you fall into the 45-54 age group, I recommend taking half a tablet (1.5 mg) before you go to bed at night. If you are between 55 and 65, you can take a full tablet, if half doesn't do the trick. And folks over 65 can take as much as two tablets.

Other conditions, such -as jet lag, insomnia, and birth control, require a different schedule. For this and other details, you should read *The Melatonin Miracle* (by Pierpaoli and Regelson, Simon and Schuster, ISBN 0-684-81335-1).

2. If it's going to make you sleepy, as it is supposed to do, then you should not drive a vehicle or operate machinery immediately after taking melatonin. This is the same advice you would receive (or should receive) if you are prescribed Valium, phenobarbital, or any other calming or sleep-inducing agent.

3. You can purchase melatonin from most health food stores or you can order Melatonin Plus from Healthy Resolve. The Healthy Resolve formula contains another excellent sleep aid called kava kava, a natural tranquilizer from the South Pacific that works well with melatonin. There is another excellent natural soporific you may want to try called valerian. But it smells like old rotten tennis shoes and, although you may actually *like* the smell of old rotten tennis shoes, most people don't.

The Human Growth Hormone

Never in my wildest dreams would I have thought, even as recently as five years ago, that I would be recommending the human growth hormone (HGH), which is secreted by the pituitary gland, for adult use. As far as our watch dogs in the PDA are concerned, it's only approved for the treatment of retarded growth in children.

But they are wrong as usual and HGH is the most exciting finding in the field of anti-aging that has thus far been discovered. That's a big claim, but the research is there and I have no doubt that HGH is the find of the century for stopping, and even reversing, the aging process. (Because of the importance of this hormone to your health and longevity, you'll want to know that it's a single chain peptide of 21,500 daltons with a sequence of 191 amino acids.)

My publisher and my editor always get a little critical with me when I discuss something that patients can't easily get. Well I understand that but, in this case, we've got to discuss it because it's too important to ignore. And it *can* be obtained — all it takes / is time and money.

One of the problems with the use of HGH has been that researchers thought they needed to use large doses as in growth retardation for an effect. This was the problem we had with chelation therapy 40 years ago when the pioneers in the field were using doses four times what was needed. As a result, some patients had serious toxicity, especially with the kidneys. It gave chelation a bad name that took many years to overcome. Today's critics, mostly out of ignorance of modern developments, but some out of a desire to sabotage chelation at any cost, cite the 40-year-old cases as if they were still valid.

This same attitude, for the same two reasons, will undoubtedly plague doctors using human growth hormone. It *was* a dangerous product as originally used, as it was obtained from cadavers and caused some fatal infections in children. And because of the very large doses they were using, as much as *15 times* the doses we use today, some patients developed diabetes, heart attacks, and infections due to a depression of the immune system. But the modern product is made by the process of genetic engineering and is completely safe, so don't let horror stories based on 50-year-old medicine, where inappropriate doses and a very inferior product were used, frighten you out of taking HGH if lab studies indicate that you need it. It can dramatically change your life — for the better.

Mild side effects may occur, but they are transient and due to the rehydration of tissues. This may crowd joints and nerves a bit causing a temporary discomfort, but it is a good sign, not a bad one. The shots are taken four times a week with a tiny needle into the skin. It's the same as taking an insulin shot and almost anyone can learn to do it.

There is no doubt that the blood level of your HGH is related to your age — the higher your age, the lower your HGH. In some elderly patients, no HGH can be detected *at all*. (I wonder if it will relieve insomnia? I've seen nothing in the literature except general references to better sleep. It may be, in conjunction with melatonin, the answer for insomnia among the elderly.)

Doctors and scientists assumed that since this hormone was so important to growth it had no further use in the body after adolescence and growth is completed. No one seemed to notice that HGH continued to hang around, although at a lower blood level, after growth was completed. Nature just doesn't work the way we think it should sometimes. If it didn't have a purpose, it would disappear from the blood. While it is true that the blood level of HGH at age 60 is only 25 percent of what it was at age 20, *it is still there*. The reason it is still there is because HGH has *profound metabolic effects* far beyond its function as a growth stimulator in the young.

As with testosterone and DHEA therapy, the objective is to get your blood levels of HGH up to that of a 20- or 30-year-old. The test used is called the IGF-1, which stands for insulin-like growth factor-one. Don't worry about the technology; just remember that the magic number for this test is 500 (units per liter) or better. Most people 60 years of age will be around 350 or lower.[1] They are shrinking and dying at a fairly steady rate. They are springing leaks, shriveling their livers and their thymus glands, and plugging arteries —

---

[1] This number will vary depending on the units of measurement the lab uses; it may be higher or lower than those numbers above. The point to remember is that you want a level that is comparable to a 20- or 30-year-old. The lab will usually report the expected range for various age groups along with the report.

they're on Nursing Home Avenue and it's a one way street —
unless they get proper hormone therapy and get it fast.

One of the interesting effects of HGH is its ability to
make a patient look remarkably younger. This may sound like
a claim from a pyramid sales organization, but there is a
good scientific reason why HGH really *is* a promoter of a
more youthful appearance. As one ages, the tissues become
desiccated; they dry up like a prune. Swedish doctors have
estimated that patients with a low HGH level can have a
body-water deficit as high as *six pints!*

The skin is no exception and so the wrinkling of the skin
is partly due to a lack of water in the deeper layers. HGH
restores the tissue water content — and thus takes 20 years off
your appearance. The protein content of tissues is also
increased by HGH, so there are really two reasons why HGH
can give you back your youthful skin.

This "youth-enhancing" effect is reason alone for most
people over 50 to want to take human growth hormone, but
the benefits go much deeper than that. The scientific
literature is replete with the remarkable attributes of this
hormone, which (until recently) was considered to be of very
limited use. After all, why would you want to give a
hormone that causes growth to someone who is already
grown and is, in fact, growing old? It just shows how a label
can cover over your whole brain and stop the reasoning
process, if you are not careful. If we had known in 1921 when
HGH was discovered that this steroid had multiple functions
and it had been called GYMH — Growth and Youth-
Maintenance Hormone — instead of Human Growth
Hormone, you would probably still be enjoying the company
of your grandparents.

Adding to the youthful appearance due to smoother
skin is the action of HGH on the distribution of body fat, the
burning off of fat and an increase of muscle mass. And this

occurs without dieting or increasing exercise. Dieting and mild exercise may improve your looks even more, but the action of HGH is independent of these.

Some scientists have suggested that obesity itself causes a depression of HGH, so simply dieting will raise the HGH level and thus obviate the need for the hormone. These critics have not thought it through. First, not all patients with a low HGH are fat, although they are likely to have the "middle-age spread" characterized by the tube around the middle. And, secondly, dieting *increases* wrinkles, those "medals of aging,"[5] rather than decreasing them. Dieting causes a generalized weight loss. You may lose fat around the middle, but you will also lose it in your face, the buttocks, and your breasts. Maybe you don't want to lose weight in all those areas.

Daniel Rudman, M.D., Medical College of Wisconsin, and his many collaborators became pioneers in the field of HGH therapy with the publication of their landmark article in the *New England Journal of Medicine* in 1990. They startled the medical world by claiming age-inhibiting properties for human growth hormone, a hormone that "everyone" knew had no further use after puberty and growth completion.

Twelve elderly men, a small study to be sure, were tested with moderately small doses of HGH and compared with nine placebo cases that were given dummy shots. Although the study group was small, the results were very impressive as compared to the men not receiving the HGH.

Here are the conclusions of the Rudman group that, at least temporarily, got the attention of the scientific community:

After six months of treatment, the HGH-treated group showed:

* an 8.8 percent increase in lean body mass (primarily muscle)

* a 14.4 percent decrease in "adipose-tissue mass" (fat)

* a 1.6 percent average increase in the density of the bones of the back (lumbar spine), i.e., less osteoporosis.
* an increase of 7.1 percent in the thickness of the skin.

Other studies quickly followed that confirmed the Rudman findings and added even more. A study from England added the following attributes to HGH therapy:

* exercise capacity "increased significantly"
* increased cardiac contractility (a stronger beating heart)
* possible increase in longevity
* a confirmation of the Rudman findings

It is said to be "normal" to deteriorate with age. Getting older is obviously not preventable, except by accident or suicide, but now, with the advent of HGH, DHEA, and the other hormonal therapies discussed here, much of the associated deterioration *is* preventable.

Let's look at two cases from the files of Dr. Elmer Cranton, who has had extensive experience with HGH therapy.

H.T., a 64-year-old businessman: H.T. has been taking HGH by injection for four years. "My energy, stamina, and sex drive are like a 30-year-old. Muscle tone is fantastically improved. My waist went down from 42 inches to 34 and I went from 29 percent fat to 12 percent. I look in the mirror in the morning and I can't believe that guy is me — it looks like me when I was 30. The palsy in my hand is gone, I discarded my bifocal glasses, and my skin went from tissue-thin to youthful."

J.H., a 40-year-old businesswoman: J.H. suffered for many years from chronic fatigue syndrome and constant pain in her jaw and head from degeneration in the jaw joint (TMJ syndrome). After taking daily HGH injections, she stated: "I was a 40-year-old woman with a 60-year-old body. On growth-hormone therapy my TMJ pain is gone completely; my energy and stamina are increased; my fat is decreased and I feel much more alive, blossoming inside, almost euphoric."

For effectiveness in using HGH, it is essential to have adequate insulin, zinc, and thyroid in your system. If you are taking a good multimineral/vitamin supplement, you are probably getting enough zinc.

Your thyroid can be checked by the underarm temperature method. Your wholistic doctor can advise you on this simple procedure.

Your doctor can check your fasting blood insulin level. Human growth hormone is usually taken in the evening and it would be good to know what your level of insulin is at your time of retiring. This is not easy to determine, but it can be worked out: Get a fasting blood insulin at your doctor's office in the morning. It won't be *exactly* the same, but if it reveals a very low blood insulin, you might benefit from a tiny dose of insulin added to the HGH shot. Insulin definitely enhances the effect of HGH. The dose of insulin we are referring to here is very small and is not dangerous.

Thymosin

As often happens in scientific research, another scientific group from across the Atlantic ocean was concurrently studying HGH, but in relation to another endocrine (glandular) system — the mysterious thymus gland and the hormone, thymosin. There are four thymic hormones. (The four thymic hormones, which interrelate in a yet undetermined manner, are: thymomodulin, thymostimulin, thymosin alpha 1 and THF — thymic humoral factor.)

This gland, located under the breast bone in front of the lungs, manufactures the T cells needed to fight infection and cancer; it is a vital part of your immune system. In the newborn, the gland is quite large and, in fact, can be so big as to cover a large part of the front of the chest. This is perfectly normal, but doctors, being doctors, over reacted with their new toy, the X-ray machine, and assumed that these large thymi were abnormal and so they proceeded to irradiate them. They had found something new to treat. They did irreparable harm to these babies, but the procedure continued for many years.

The thymus shrinks in childhood, and later in life it is often hard to find at all. This is very puzzling because there is no doubt of the importance of the gland. Why does it practically disappear? How do we manage to live without it?

The thymus continues to fascinate scientists and, while Rudman was reporting on the general physiological effects of HGH, Italian investigators were reporting in the journal, *Hormone Research*, on the effect of HGH on the thymus gland. They were able to show that HGH has a direct stimulating action on the thymus causing a significant rise in blood thymosin levels after a single injection. European doctors have been prescribing thymus shots for years, but as HGH will stimulate the thymus directly, and HGH has so many other benefits, HGH therapy is perhaps a better way.

A Summary on the Benefits of HGH

There are so many facets to the HGH story, so many ways that it can improve your health, that a summary of the functions of this incredible hormone from the pituitary is in order. Tissue repair, healing, cell replacement, organ repair (such as the liver and brain), bone strength, enzyme production, and the integrity of hair, nails, and skin all require adequate amounts of growth hormone on a regular basis. Learning, memory, and intelligence all depend on adequate HGH levels and these important aspects of a truly happy old age are denied to many because of HGH deficiency.

54

Scientifically proven benefits of HGH therapy include increased muscle mass, increased physical strength, reduced fatigue, decreased fat, increased bone strength, and a revitalization of all the body's organs — liver, kidney, spleen, and brain, to name a few. The skin improves dramatically and sexual function increases. Cholesterol decreases and some of our most dreaded diseases are improved by HGH: Alzheimer's disease, osteoporosis, and Parkinson's disease. It improves, but does not cure, AIDS.

An important aspect of HGH therapy is the enhancement of the immune system, which opens the avenue to the treatment of another host of man's worst problems: infections (now going out of control), allergies, arthritis, and cancer. So now perhaps you can see why I call the advent of HGH treatment the single most important advance in anti-aging therapy in medical history.

Thyroid Hormone — Thyroxin

In a simplistic way, aging seems to be a string of hormone deficiencies, from melatonin to growth hormone to thyroid and on down the body to testosterone and the other sex hormones. Thyroid hormone, thyroxin, is probably the most "recognized" of the hormones, but it is also the most poorly treated, at least in its deficiency state: hypothyroidism.

Many patients are confused as to whether low thyroid is called hyper or hypo so they mumble something like "hymmmthyroidism." People don't like to admit ignorance, even to their doctor. Let's settle this once and for all — hypo means low (it rhymes) so we are talking about hypothyroidism. (Hyper, overactive thyroid, is hyperthyroidism. We are not going to spend any time on the hyperactive stage of thyroid disease because, unfortunately, those of us in alternative medicine can't treat it effectively. I wish we could treat it, because the conventional docs don't do all that well treating it either.)

One of the greatest errors in medicine today is the treating of hypothyroidism with something that isn't thyroid. Just like the doctors have been treating low estrogen states ("menopause") and low progesterone states ("PMS") with synthetic hormones, they use a synthetic thyroid that isn't thyroid and a large proportion of patients simply don't respond. I'd like to have a hundred dollar bill for every patient I have taken off Synthroid, the synthetic, and placed on natural thyroid, often with a dramatic improvement.

I've told you many times that misdiagnosis is a major reason some people never recover from an illness. If a disease is misdiagnosed, it will probably be mistreated. And now, a report from England again illustrates this and shows why you (and your grandma) should patronize a wholistic physician.

A woman in late middle age became lethargic, stooped, and generally uninterested in life. While most doctors would have diagnosed this gentle lady with Alzheimer's, she actually suffered from hypothyroidism (low thyroid production).

Fortunately for her, an alert doctor did not assume that she had Alzheimer's disease, although she was precisely at the age for its onset and looked like a "classic" case. After being put on a small dose of natural thyroid, "she was back at work, studying for an Open University degree, and riding her bike."

And this is not a rare case. Hospitals, private homes, and nursing facilities are full of tragedies like this.

Another remarkable case of undiagnosed hypothyroid-ism was reported in *Discover* magazine, February 1988, by Dr. Oliver Sacks of Albert Einstein College of Medicine.

"Uncle Toby" was a modern-day Rip van Winkle. He sat in a chair for *seven years* hardly moving. He was fed and watered like a plant.

Dr. Sacks, while on a house call, noticed Uncle Toby sitting in the corner and inquired as to his problem. The family said he had been that way since 1950 — out to lunch — in a deep freeze. He was just a piece of furniture that was rearranged occasionally.

Toby was admitted to the hospital and was found to have essentially zero thyroid function. His temperature was 68 degrees Fahrenheit! (Ninety-six degrees would be considered clear evidence of hypothyroidism.)

After treatment, Uncle Toby came to and had no awareness of having lost seven years of his life.

Another case of hypothyroidism successfully treated by Dr. Sacks was misdiagnosed so badly that he had undergone psychiatric treatment, with tranquilizers, for 29 years.

Well informed wholistic physicians have been aware of chronic thyroid deficiency, especially in the elderly, for 40 years and have been treating it with cow- or pork-based natural thyroid. The uptown endocrinologists have always scoffed at this therapy. But the patient whose tests indicate that thyroid function is normal and isn't happy with the inevitable tranquilizer therapy should look for a good quack who really understands thyroid. A doctor who understands thyroid can often work miracles, even when the blood tests indicate that thyroid function is normal.

Just to give you some idea of the catholicity of this problem, here are just a few of the symptoms that this hormone deficiency can cause: dryness of the hair and skin; fatigue; inability to concentrate; memory loss; cold intolerance; swelling of the face, hands, and feet; irritability; depression; decreased sex drive; anxiety; hair loss; obesity, (actually fluid retention and not true fatness — a patient can be severely hypothyroid and be underweight); and an Alzheimer-like condition, as with Uncle Toby.

The nursing homes are warehousing many of these unfortunate, undiagnosed cases of hypothyroidism. And most doctors, even if they suspect a low thyroid in an elderly patient, will prescribe a synthetic hormone, called Synthroid, because the drug salesman told him that this ersatz form of thyroid was better, i.e., more pure, more predictable, more consistent, more effective, etc. — none of which are true.

I remember vividly the first time a "detail man" (pharmaceutical salesman) came into my office to sell me on his synthetic thyroid hormone. I was fresh out of the U.S. Navy and naive enough to think that the drug pushers representing the pharmaceutical industry would help me practice better medicine. He said the synthetic hormone was better than the natural variety because it represented a pure chemical and so was uniform and more predictable in response. (Homogenized milk is more uniform, too, and it hardens your arteries.)

The salesman's pitch for Synthroid sounded convincing because I was inexperienced in the treatment of hypothyroidism. It wasn't until a few years later that I became aware as to why the synthetic thyroid often didn't work. Synthetic thyroid hormone is called T-4. Natural thyroid is T-3. Synthroid has to be converted from T-4 to T-3 by the body in order to be utilized. Many people suffering from hypothyroidism cannot make this conversion.

But most hypothyroid patients never even get the opportunity to fail on the synthetic *as they don't get treated at all.* This is because most doctors don't know how to test properly for low thyroid function. One needs to go "low tech" when testing for this disease. The expensive laboratory tests are not accurate enough to pick up subclinical cases of hypothyroidism. ("Subclinical" means the disease is there, but the doctor hasn't been clever enough to make the diagnosis.)

The most common complaints associated with hypothyroidism are fatigue and intolerance to cold. If you are shivering and everyone else is comfortable, you are probably thyroid deficient. There can be an almost infinite variety of complaints associated with hypothyroidism from mental aberrations to constipation, from skin problems to heart manifestations and sexual dysfunction. The reason for this variety of infirmities is because *thyroid hormone is essential for the healthy function of every cell in your body.*

A simple morning temperature test that you can do at home is better than all the fancy and expensive lab tests combined. Millions of dollars are wasted every year on thyroid tests that usually don't reveal a low-functioning thyroid unless you are half dead, like Uncle Toby. So many people drag themselves through life not getting thyroid supplementation that they desperately need because the doctors relied on inaccurate lab testing.

To do the thyroid test, place a thermometer next to your bed (shake it down to 95 before you go to sleep). The next morning, put the thermometer in your arm pit firmly and leave it there for three minutes. *Lie still* because activity will raise your temperature and give a deceptively high reading. Do the test for a couple of days to confirm the readings. If the temperature is consistently 97.8 or lower, you are thyroid deficient and you should see a qualified physician for treatment. *If you have a cold,* or other illness, or you are in the last two weeks of your menstrual cycle, wait until you are well, or post-menstrual, before doing the series of temperature readings.

The hypothyroid story has proven to be more extensive than even those of us who practice natural thyroid medicine had known. Dr. David S. Cooper of Johns Hopkins University says that 15 percent of women and eight percent of men over 60 suffer from low thyroid function. After many years of checking people for this condition, I think it is even more common than that. We even see thyroid deficiency in children. I think 50 percent of people over 50 suffer from some degree of hypothyroidism.

Thyroid doesn't just give the patient energy and increased mental awareness. Somehow, the thyroid hormone protects the heart. People with overactive thyroid glands –

thyroidism rarely have heart attacks. Thyroid is also ful in the treatment of premenstrual syndrome. Every oman suffering from premenstrual syndrome should take the temperature test and take thyroid if the test so indicates.

Iodine is the key element that is essential for the body to manufacture the thyroid hormone in the thyroid gland. We used to think that hypothyroidism was due to iodine-deficient soil, which produces iodine-deficient vegetables. But we see hypothyroidism in all areas of the country, so there has to be another explanation.

I think it's due to drinking chlorinated, fluoridated water. Chlorine, fluorine, and iodine are chemical triplets. They only differ in their atomic weight. The chlorine, and/or fluorine probably blocks the iodine receptor sites on the thyroid gland thus making it impossible for the gland to receive and utilize this vital element. With people restricting their salt intake, which is usually "iodized," they have even *less* iodine to compete with the chlorine and fluorine in the water they drink. This salt restriction is often the result of bad advice from a doctor.

It is important that you go to a doctor who *really understands* how to use natural thyroid. It *is* more unpredictable than the synthetics because it is four times more potent and longer acting than the synthetic chemical. It is amazing that so many people are taking natural thyroid with little medical supervision and they seldom get into trouble with it. Theoretically, they should have overdose complications occasionally, but most do not. But if *you* are one of the unfortunate ones who does get an overdose reaction, you are not going to be comforted by the statistic that *most* people do not experience an overdose. Follow the advice of your wholistic doctor.

There is a simple answer to this dilemma and that is for the doctor to have the pharmacist compound a long-acting preparation that will give a smooth release of the hormone and thus avoid any ups and downs in dosage. The only problem is the PDA is going to decree that all compounds the doctor orders the pharmacist to make for his patients are illegal because they are "new drugs" and haven't been approved by his betters in the bureaucracy.

Anyway, you must use natural thyroid as long as it is legal. Don't worry about the irregularity thing too much. You are not going to kill yourself. If you develop symptoms of too much thyroid (nervousness, sleeplessness, palpitations, diarrhea) see your natural thyroid doctor and he will adjust the dosage. While you're there, ask your doctor if you need iodine supplementation. Iodine can sometimes have remarkable positive effects on many diseases, including cystic breast disease.

I once had a patient who had to take *12 grains a day of natural thyroid* in order to function well. That is *12 times* the usual daily dose. An endocrinologist told her it was dangerous quackery and that it was going to kill her. Frightened half to death, she stopped taking any thyroid and considered charging me with attempted murder. *He* almost killed her as she went into a severe myxedema crisis where everything shut down. She said she knew she was dying (and I think she was right). After going back on her 12 grains of thyroid a day, she was completely normal again.

ACE:
The Next Hormone Therapy?

We have by no means covered all of the hormones in this report, or even all of the important ones. We haven't mentioned parahormone, ACTH, FSH, LH, TSH, ADH and many, many others. What we have presented here are the hormones that we know can offer you better health and increased longevity *now*. Modern medicine is largely a "seek and destroy" system, a desperation mind-set that attacks disease with chemicals and extirpative surgery (the surgeons have a motto: "When in doubt, cut it out") and has little or no thought for prevention. These hormone therapies are both curative and preventive.

By now, it should be obvious to you that the conventional medical profession is missing the boat on the hormone revolution. The question is why? You have probably guessed the answer: Most of the treatments described in this report are basic, generic hormones that carry little profit potential. So the drug companies and the medical journals are not going to spend time and money reminding doctors of therapeutic agents in which there is no profit.

A good example of this suppression of an excellent, safe hormone by the pharmaceutical / governmental cabal is Adrenal Cortical Extract — ACE. Many of us in the wholistic field of medicine used ACE with great success for many years in a broad spectrum of diseases. It contained all of the life-sustaining hormones of the adrenal cortex and could be given with complete confidence in its safety, when used properly. For fatigue, "adrenal exhaustion" (not easy to confirm by conventional laboratory tests) and chronic fatigue syndrome, nothing works better than adrenal cortical extract injections (one or two mis given monthly or more often according to the response).

The reason for its effectiveness is that ACE is a combination of many of the most important hormones in the body. Sugar, sodium, potassium, and all the sex hormones are controlled by the hormones from the adrenal cortex. There is no system that is not influenced by the hormones of the adrenal "cortex" (the outer layers of the adrenal glands, which sit on top of the kidneys).

It's interesting to note that chronic fatigue syndrome became recognized as a disease state (at least by doctors in the field of alternative medicine) just about the time that the PDA began to intimidate the small companies that were making ACE available to us. The geniuses of the PDA said that adrenal cortical extract was no longer necessary as all the hormones it contained were now available in synthetic form (not true) and so treatment could be more specific, aimed at the deficiency present in each patient (as if doctors were smart enough to know exactly what the patient needed).

So ACE disappeared from the market and chronic fatigue syndrome became one of the mystery diseases of the late 20th century. I am not implying that the loss of ACE led to the increase of chronic fatigue syndrome, but if ACE had not been denied to us, I really believe a lot of suffering could have been avoided.

While ACE might have been pulled off the shelves, I don't think the hormone revolution can be stopped. We are facing a sea change in longevity and health in the elderly and as the baby boomer generation slips past middle age, the time has never been riper for hormone therapy.

Henry Wordsworth Longfellow tried to console us in our declining, so-called golden years, when everything is falling apart and we have aches from here to there:

> For age is opportunity no less
> Than youth itself, though in another dress,
> And as the evening twilight fades away
> The sky is filled by stars, invisible by day.

That's really a beautiful poem. But with due regard for Henry, most of us would like to be able to *see* the stars, *walk* in the twilight unassisted, and *smell* the roses — and we would also like to live just a wee bit longer. The really good news is that our ability to influence longevity is growing. And hormone therapy is just the beginning. Now that you've read about all the benefits this revolution is bringing to us, I

63

think you'll agree that the golden years can be some of the most productive years of your life. Yes, indeed, aging is an opportunity — and no less.

If you want more information or need help finding a doctor that's familiar with hormone therapy replacement, contact the folks at Broda O. Barnes Research Foundation (P.O. Box 98, Trumbill, CT 06611, 203-261-2101). These wonderful people should be able to help you with any questions you might have. And the doctors they recommend will usually understand all the hormonal problems mentioned in this monograph, as well as the proper methods for treating them.

WHY YOU DON'T NEED A MAMMOGRAM

If you're an American woman, you're at risk from breast cancer. "One in nine" is the frightening statistic released by the National Cancer Institute (NCI), which started aggressively publicizing breast cancer rates back in 1970 — when the figure was one in 16 —as a way to scare women into the doctor's office.

Women, horrified by pictures of the mutilating effects of uncaring and condescending doctors, responded in droves to the NCI's demand for regular breast checkups and mammograms. The campaign has been so successful (and a cash cow) that today, you can even call a roaming mobile mammography unit to your front door for an onthe-spot screening!

Prevention like this seems a logical weapon against this cancerous killer. But in fact, we are now beginning to see examples of *tests* for cancer actually increasing the *incidence* of cancer. I've been warning women for years that annual mammographic screening of women without symptoms may produce more cancer than it detects.

The National "Canard" Institute

The NCI conducted a study of the effectiveness of cancer screening and detection. Their report was a classic example of government double-talk and institutionalized disregard for women.

Although the breast cancer detection rate is the "highest on record," we are experiencing "the highest incidence rates (of breast cancer) ever recorded." In 10 years there

65

has been a 17 percent increase in breast cancer despite massive public education campaigns and a consequent dramatic increase in the number of women screened.

Then the NCI's report went on to wail that "little effective screening is taking place." Early detection through mammography, they said, "can reduce the mortality rate from (breast cancer) by more than 30 percent."

Then why hasn't it? The mortality rate has gone up instead of down!

What's next?

The latest shocker has to do with the highly-touted X-ray mammography. Women are constantly reassured that mammograms are safe "because the amount of radiation is very small." But this reassurance completely overlooks a serious problem with mammography. Sometimes it's not an "overlook" but an complete disregard for the danger involved when the procedure is not performed carefully.

Although widely used for early cancer detection screening, remarkably little attention has been paid to the techniques of breast compression used in the mammography procedure. It is generally accepted that any cancer should be handled as carefully as possible, with very gentle palpation, in order to avoid accidental spread of the disease. As long ago as 1928, Dr. D.T. Quigley warned of the dangers of rough treatment of breast cancers.

Although the principle of gentle handling of cancer is widely accepted, when it comes to testing for the disease, all logic seems to go out the window and the handling of tissues, such as the female breast, gets very rough indeed. We're not talking Lothario here, rather doctors who see breasts as sacks of money to be milked, rather than fountains of nourishment for the nation's babies and lovely symbols of the female gender.

Ouch!

Techniques used are designed for maximum detection of cancerous tissue without regard for the possible disastrous consequences. One survey found that the mammographers used "as much compression as the patient could tolerate"—and had no idea how much compression they were actually using. As the guidelines state, for proper mammography, "adequacy of the compression device is crucial to good quality mammography." In other words, squeeze the hell out of the breast for clear pictures and just forget about the Hippocratic admonition to do the patient no harm. As a mammographer, you must have good pictures. If you miss a cancer, you'll get sued. So the patient isn't the only one who can get squeezed.

The recommended force to be used in order to compress the breast tissue enough for a proper mammogram is 300 newtons. That's the equivalent of 50 pounds of pressure on the breast.

As so often happens in clinical medicine, the practice of the art is often not consistent with the findings of science. One animal study found that the number of metastases (or, spread of a cancer) will increase by eighty percent if the tumor is manipulated. A human study reported in the British MedicalJournal confirms these ominous findings. They discovered there were 29 percent more deaths from breast cancer in women who had mammograms.

It's mammography, stupid!

A report from the National Cancer Institute of Canada was interesting in that it completely missed the point on why cancer seems to be higher in women who take their doctor's advice and get mammograms. They reported, as in the above study, that women who have regular mammograms are more likely to die of breast cancer than women who eschew this test. But the investigators didn't blame the mammography procedure itself for the bad results they found and instead blamed "modern treatment."

Professor Anthony Miller of the Toronto University Medical School, who was director of the study said, "You may find the cancer earlier but the women are still going to die. Modern treatment does not work for these early cancers."

While I agree completely with Dr. Miller's assessment of modern cancer therapy, it is unfortunate that their study was blind to the danger of the mammography procedure itself.

A British surgeon, Dr. Baum, says screening women under 50 was "opportunistic" and did more harm than good. He also said that "99.85 percent of premenopausal women will have no benefit from screening. Even for women over 50, there has been only a one percent biopsy rate as a result of screening in the U.K."

Doctor's orders

Keeping all of the above in mind, here are my recommendations:

1) First of all look at the NCI's ominous statistic, one in nine, more closely (which they don't want you to do) and you'll see that the average woman has an *89 percent* chance of **never** developing breast cancer.

2) Stay away from so-called anticancer drugs. None of them work for cancer of the breast (and they'll probably cause some unwanted and dangerous side effects, too).

3) Stay away from the estrogens so many physicians are pushing to reduce symptoms of menopause.

Menopausal symptoms, like hot flashes, will clear up within a year if nature is allowed to take its course. It is clear these estrogens are causing cancer of the breast. Dr. Robert Hoover of the National Cancer Institute said: "The fact that ovarian hormones might relate to increased risk of breast cancer is not on the bizarre fringe of biological reasoning. The biological plausibility was established 100 years ago, so new data which shows that women on (estrogen) replacement therapy have an increased risk [of cancer] is exactly what you would predict."

4) Examine your breasts once a month (a week after your period—lumps are not unusual the week before). If something seems abnormal to you, go see your doctor. Odds are greatly in your favor that the lump you have discovered is benign.

5) Don't get a mammogram at the drop of a hat. My position used to be, the test won't hurt you but it may encourage a surgeon to do surgery that will shorten your life, not to mention the threat of chemotherapy. But now it is clear that the test itself is dangerous and may spread cancer even faster than the surgeon.

6) But if the doctor is persistent, wait a month before doing anything. Time is not the important factor. It may take a fly speck-sized cancer 10 or 20 years to grow to the size of a walnut. Early surgery and radiation may stimulate rather than cure the cancer. With earlier 'treatment' it becomes a contest as to which will kill the patient, the treatment or the cancer.

7) On reexamination, if the lump is larger, and did not recede after your period, then ask for an excisional biopsy (a "lumpectomy"). Do not let him do a needle biopsy. I have said for years that a needle biopsy is

69

tantamount to cutting through a cancer—something doctors try to avoid during surgery. Putting a needle into the cancer is just like cutting into it with a tiny knife, and recent studies have shown that cancer cells do indeed migrate along the path of the needle.

8) Do not submit to more surgery than a simple lump removal. In a study involving 259 women in nine medical centers, it was shown that a simple lumpectomy offers as long a survival time as a radical mastectomy. In many cases, survival is longer. The study included radiation therapy along with the simple lumpectomy. Next they will find that the radiation is not necessary and is probably contraindicated. But that will take another 20 years.

9) Do not allow them to cut into the lymph nodes in your arm pit.

Approximately 30 percent of women whose axillary lymph nodes appear disease-free at surgery eventually develop metastases or a new cancer in other breast. The NCI's answer? They recommend that all breast cancer patients receive chemotherapy (which doesn't work on cancer).

10) Pass on the radiation and chemotherapy. Radiation is highly destructive of not only tissues, but the immune system, which then makes you more susceptible to all diseases. It is usually a terrible price to pay for a temporary shrinkage of a tumor or to destroy "leftover" cancer cells post-surgery.

About Doctor William Campbell Douglass II

Dr. Douglass reveals medical truths, and deceptions, often at risk of being labeled heretical. He is consumed by a passion for living a long healthy life, and wants his readers to share that passion. Their health and well-being comes first. He is anti-dogmatic, and unwavering in his dedication to improve the quality of life of his readers. He has been called "the conscience of modern medicine," a "medical maverick," and has been voted "Doctor of the Year" by the National Health Federation. His medical experiences are far reaching-from battling malaria in Central America - to fighting deadly epidemics at his own health clinic in Africa - to flying with U.S. Navy crews as a flight surgeon - to working for 10 years in emergency medicine here in the States. These learning experiences, not to mention his keen storytelling ability and wit, make Dr. Douglass' newsletters (Daily Dose and Real Health) and books uniquely interesting and fun to read. He shares his no-frills, no-bull approach to health care, often amazing his readers by telling them to ignore many widely-hyped good-health practices (like staying away from red meat, avoiding coffee, and eating like a bird), and start living again by eating REAL food, taking some inexpensive supplements, and doing the pleasurable things that make life livable. Readers get all this, plus they learn how to burn fat, prevent cancer, boost libido, and so much more. And, Dr. Douglass is not afraid to challenge the latest studies that come out, and share the real story with his readers. Dr. William C. Douglass has led a colorful, rebellious, and crusading life. Not many physicians would dare put their professional reputations on the line as many times as this courageous healer has. A vocal opponent of "business-as-usual" medicine, Dr. Douglass has championed patients' rights and physician commitment to wellness throughout his career. This dedicated physician has repeatedly gone far beyond the call of duty in his work to spread the truth about alternative therapies. For a full year, he endured economic and physical hardship to work with physicians at the Pasteur Institute in St. Petersburg, Russia, where advanced research on photoluminescence was being conducted. Dr. Douglass comes from a distinguished family of physicians. He is the fourth generation Douglass to practice medicine, and his son is also a physician. Dr. Douglass graduated from the University of Rochester, the Miami School of Medicine, and the Naval School of Aviation and Space Medicine.

You want to protect those you love from the health dangers the authorities aren't telling you about, and learn the incredible cures that they've scorned and ignored?
Subscribe to the free Daily Dose updates "...the straight scoop about health, medicine, and politics." by sending an e-mail to real_sub@agoramail.net with the word "subscribe" in the subject line.

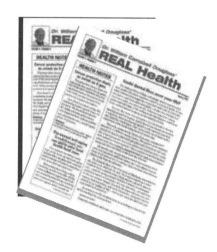

If you knew of a procedure that could save thousands, maybe millions, of people dying from AIDS, cancer, and other dreaded killers....

Would you cover it up?

It's unthinkable that what could be the best solution ever to stopping the world's killer diseases is being ignored, scorned, and rejected. But that is exactly what's happening right now.

The procedure is called "photoluminescence". It's a thoroughly tested, proven therapy that uses the healing power of the light to perform almost miraculous cures.

This remarkable treatment works its incredible cures by stimulating the body's own immune responses. That's why it cures so many ailments--and why it's been especially effective against AIDS! Yet, 50 years ago, it virtually disappeared from the halls of medicine.

Why has this incredible cure been ignored by the medical authorities of this country? You'll find the shocking answer here in the pages of this new edition of Into the Light. Now available with the blood irradiation Instrument Diagram and a complete set of instructions for building your own "Treatment Device". Also includes details on how to use this unique medical instrument.

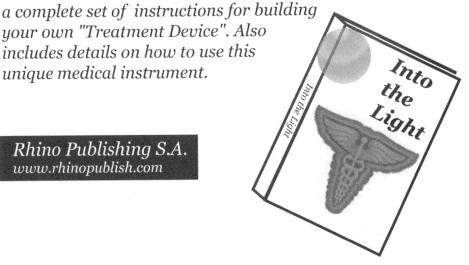

Rhino Publishing S.A.
www.rhinopublish.com

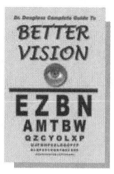

Dr. Douglass' Complete Guide to Better Vision

A report about eyesight and what can be done to improve it naturally. But I've also included information about how the eye works, brief descriptions of various common eye conditions, traditional remedies to eye problems, and a few simple suggestions that may help you maintain your eyesight for years to come.
-William Campbell Douglass II, MD

The Hypertension Report.
Say Good Bye to High Blood Pressure.

An estimated 50 million Americans have high blood pressure. Often called the "silent killer" because it may not cause symptoms until the patient has suffered serious damage to the arterial system. Diet, exercise, potassium supplements chelation therapy and practically anything but drugs is the way to go and alternatives are discussed in this report.

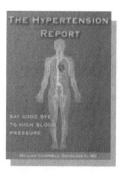

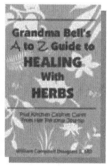

Grandma Bell's A To Z Guide To Healing With Herbs.

This book is all about - coming home. What I once believed to be old wives' tales - stories long destroyed by the new world of science - actually proved to be the best treatment for many of the common ailments you and I suffer through. So I put a few of them together in this book with the sincere hope that Grandma Bell's wisdom will help you recover your common sense, and take responsibility for your own health. -William Campbell Douglass II, MD

Prostate Problems:
Safe, Simple, Effective Relief for Men over 50.

Don't be frightened into surgery or drugs you may not need. First, get the facts about prostate problems... know all your options, so you can make the best decisions. This fully documented report explains the dangers of conventional treatments, and gives you alternatives that could save you more than just money!

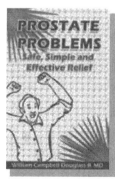

Color me Healthy
The Healing Powers
of Colors

"He's crazy!"
"He's got to be a quack!"
"Who gave this guy his medical license?"
"He's a nut case!"

In case you're wondering, those are the reactions you'll probably get if you show your doctor this report. I know the idea of healing many common ailments simply by exposing them to colored light sounds far-fetched, but when you see the evidence, you'll agree that color is truly an amazing medical breakthrough.

When I first heard the stories, I reacted much the same way. But the evidence so convinced me, that I had to try color therapy in my practice. My results were truly amazing.

-William Campbell Douglass II, MD

Order your complete set of Roscolene filters (choice of 3 sizes) to be used with the "Color Me Healthy" therapy. The eleven Roscolene filters are # 809, 810, 818, 826, 828, 832, 859, 861, 866, 871, and 877. The filters come with protective separator sheets between each filter. The color names and the Roscolene filter(s) used to produce that particular color, are printed on a card included with the filters and a set of instructions on how to fit them to a lamp.

What Is Going on Here?

Peroxides are supposed to be bad for you. Free radicals and all that. But now we hear that hydrogen peroxide is good for us. Hydrogen peroxide will put extra oxygen in your blood. There's no doubt about that. Hydrogen peroxide costs pennies. So if you can get oxygen into the blood cheaply and safely, maybe cancer (which doesn't like oxygen), emphysema, AIDS, and many other terrible diseases can be treated effectively. Intravenous hydrogen peroxide rapidly relieves allergic reactions, influenza symptoms, and acute viral infections.

No one expects to live forever. But we would all like to have a George Burns finish. The prospect of finishing life in a nursing home after abandoning your tricycle in the mobile home park is not appealing. Then comes the loss of control of vital functions the ultimate humiliation. Is life supposed to be from tricycle to tricycle and diaper to diaper? You come into this world crying, but do you have to leave crying? I don't believe you do. And you won't either after you see the evidence. Sounds too good to be true, doesn't it? Read on and decide for yourself.

-William Campbell Douglass II, MD

Rhino Publishing S.A.
www.rhinopublish.com

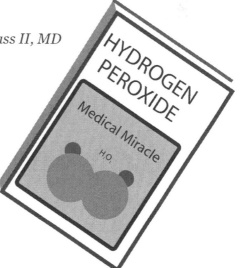

Don't drink your milk!

If you knew what we know about milk... BLEECHT! All that pasteurization, homogenization and processing is not only cooking all the nutrients right out of your favorite drink. It's also adding toxic levels of vitamin D.

This fascinating book tells the whole story about milk. How it once was nature's perfect food...how "raw," unprocessed milk can heal and boost your immune system ... why you can't buy it legally in this country anymore, and what we could do to change that.

Dr. "Douglass traveled all over the world, tasting all kinds of milk from all kinds of cows, poring over dusty research books in ancient libraries far from home, to write this light-hearted but scientifically sound book.

Rhino Publishing, S.A.
www.rhinopublish.com

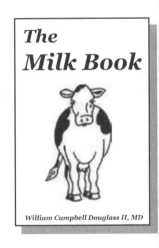

The Milk Book

William Campbell Douglass II, MD

Eat Your Cholesterol!

Eat Meat, Drink Milk, Spread The Butter- And Live Longer!
How to Live off the Fat of the Land and Feel Great.

Americans are being saturated with anti-cholesterol propaganda. If you watch very much television, you're probably one of the millions of Americans who now has a terminal case of cholesterol phobia. The propaganda is relentless and is often designed to produce fear and loathing of this worst of all food contaminants. You never hear the food propagandists bragging about their product being fluoride-free or aluminum-free, two of our truly serious food-additive problems. But cholesterol, an essential nutrient, not proven to be harmful in any quantity, is constantly pilloried as a menace to your health. If you don't use corn oil, Fleischmann's margarine, and Egg Beaters, you're going straight to atherosclerosis hell with stroke, heart attack, and premature aging -- and so are your kids. Never feel guilty about what you eat again! Dr. Douglass shows you why red meat, eggs, and dairy products aren't the dietary demons we're told they are. But beware: This scientifically sound report goes against all the "common wisdom" about the foods you should eat. Read with an open mind.

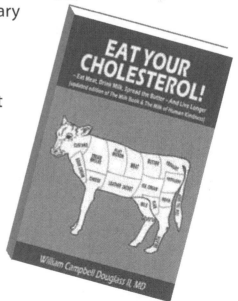

Rhino Publishing, S.A.
www.rhinopublish.com

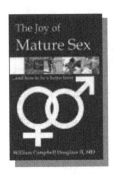

The Joy of Mature Sex and How to Be a Better Lover

Humans are very confused about what makes good sex. But I believe humans have more to offer each other than this total licentiousness common among animals. We're talking about mature sex. The kind of sex that made this country great.

Stop Aging or Slow the Process How Exercise With Oxygen Therapy (EWOT) Can Help

EWOT (pronounced ee-watt) stands for Exercise With Oxygen Therapy. This method of prolonging your life is so simple and you can do it at home at a minimal cost. When your cells don't get enough oxygen, they degenerate and die and so you degenerate and die. It's as simple as that.

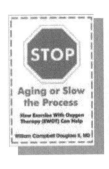

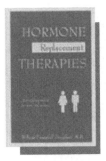

Hormone Replacement Therapies: Astonishing Results For Men And Women

It is accurate to say that when the endocrine glands start to fail, you start to die. We are facing a sea change in longevity and health in the elderly. Now, with the proper supplemental hormones, we can slow the aging process and, in many cases, reverse some of the signs and symptoms of aging.

Add 10 Years to Your Life With some "best of" Dr. Douglass' writings.

To add ten years to your life, you need to have the right attitude about health and an understanding of the health industry and what it's feeding you. Following the established line on many health issues could make you very sick or worse! Achieve dynamic health with this collection of some of the "best of" Dr. Douglass' newsletters.

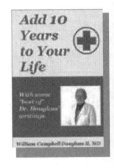

How did AIDS become one of the Greatest Biological Disasters in the History of Mankind?

GET THE FACTS

AIDS and BIOLOGICAL WARFARE covers the history of plagues from the past to today's global confrontation with AIDS, the Prince of Plagues. Completely documented *AIDS and BIOLOGICAL WARFARE* helps you make your own decisions about how to survive in a world ravaged by this horrible plague.

You will learn that AIDS is not a naturally occuring disease process as you have been led to believe, but a man-made biological nightmare that has been unleashed and is now threatening the very existence of human life on the planet.

There is a smokescreen of misinformation clouding the AIDS issue. Now, for the first time, learn the truth about the nature of the crisis our planet faces: its origin -- how AIDS is really transmited and alternatives for treatment. Find out what they are not telling you about AIDS and Biological Warfare, and how to protect yourself and your loved ones. AIDS is a serious problem worldwide, but it is no longer the major threat. You need to know the whole story. To protect yourself, you must know the truth about biological warfare.

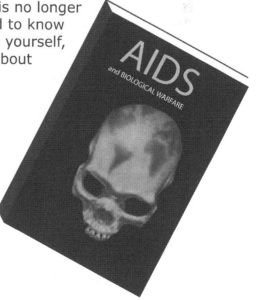

Rhino Publishing S.A.
www.rhinopublish.com

PAINFUL DILEMMA

Are we fighting the wrong war?

We are spending millions on the war against drugs while we
should be fighting the war against pain with those drugs!

As you will read in this book, the war on drugs was lost a long time ago and,
when it comes to the war against pain, pain is winning! An article in USA Today
(11/20/02) reveals that dying patients are not getting relief from pain. It seems
the doctors are torn between fear of the government, certainly justified, and a
clinging to old and out dated ideas about pain, which is NOT justified.

A group called Last Acts, a coalition of health-care groups, has released a very
discouraging study of all 50 states that nearly half of the 1.6 million Americans
living in nursing homes suffer from untreated pain. They said that life was being
extended but it amounted to little more than "extended pain and suffering."

This book offers insight into the history of pain treatment and the current failed
philosophies of contemporary medicine. Plus it describes some of today's most
advanced treatments for alleviating certain kinds of pain. This book is not another
"self-help" book touting home remedies; rather, Painful Dilemma: Patients in
Pain -- People in Prison, takes a hard look at where we've gone wrong and what
we (you) can do to help a loved one who is living with chronic pain.

The second half of this book is a must read if you value your freedom. We now
have the ridiculous and tragic situation of people
in pain living in a government-created hell by
restriction of narcotics and people in prison for
trying to bring pain relief by the selling of
narcotics to the suffering. The end result of the
"war on drugs" has been to create the greatest
and most destructive cartel in history, so great,
in fact, that the drug Mafia now controls most
of the world economy.

PAINFUL DILEMMA
PATIENTS IN PAIN
PEOPLE IN PRISON

Rhino Publishing S.A.
www.rhinopublish.com

Live the Adventure!

Why would anyone in their right mind put everything they own in storage and move to Russia, of all places?! But when maverick physician Bill Douglass left a profitable medical practice in a peaceful mountaintop town to pursue "pure medical truth".... none of us who know him well was really surprised.

After All, anyone who's braved the outermost reaches of darkest Africa, the mean streets of Johannesburg and New York, and even a trip to Washington to testify before the Senate, wouldn't bat and eye at ducking behind the Iron Curtain for a little medical reconnaissance!

Enjoy this imaginative, funny, dedicated man's tales of wonder and woe as he treks through a year in St. Petersburg, working on a cure for the world's killer diseases. We promise --

YOU WON'T BE BORED!

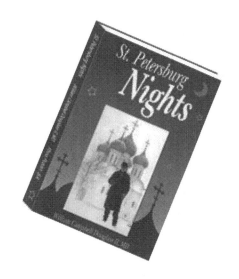

Rhino Publishing S.A.
www.rhinopublish.com

THE SMOKER'S PARADOX
THE HEALTH BENEFITS OF TOBACCO!

The benefits of smoking tobacco have been common knowledge for centuries. From sharpening mental acuity to maintaining optimal weight, the relatively small risks of smoking have always been outweighed by the substantial improvement to mental and physical health. Hysterical attacks on tobacco notwithstanding, smokers always weigh the good against the bad and puff away or quit according to their personal preferences. Now the same anti-tobacco enterprise that has spent billions demonizing the pleasure of smoking is providing additional reasons to smoke. Alzheimer's, Parkinson's, Tourette's Syndrome, even schizophrenia and cocaine addiction are disorders that are alleviated by tobacco. Add in the still inconclusive indication that tobacco helps to prevent colon and prostate cancer and the endorsement for smoking tobacco by the medical establishment is good news for smokers and non-smokers alike. Of course the revelation that tobacco is good for you is ruined by the pharmaceutical industry's plan to substitute the natural and relatively inexpensive tobacco plant with their overpriced and ineffective nicotine substitutions. Still, when all is said and done, the positive revelations regarding tobacco are very good reasons indeed to keep lighting those cigars - but only 4 a day!

Rhino Publishing, S.A
www.rhinopublish.com

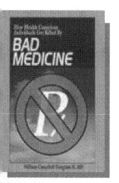

Bad Medicine
How Individuals Get Killed By Bad Medicine.

Do you really need that new prescription or that overnight stay in the hospital? In this report, Dr. Douglass reveals the common medical practices and misconceptions endangering your health. Best of all, he tells you the pointed (but very revealing!) questions your doctor prays you never ask. Interesting medical facts about popular remedies are revealed.

Dangerous Legal Drugs
The Poisons in Your Medicine Chest.

If you knew what we know about the most popular prescription and over-the-counter drugs, you'd be sick. That's why Dr. Douglass wrote this shocking report about the poisons in your medicine chest. He gives you the low-down on different categories of drugs. Everything from painkillers and cold remedies to tranquilizers and powerful cancer drugs.

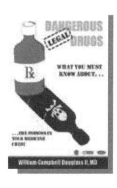

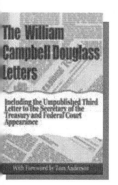

The William Campbell Douglass Letters.
Expose of Government Machinations
(Vietnam War).

THE WILLIAM CAMPBELL DOUGLASS LETTERS. Dr. Douglass' Defense in 1968 Tax Case and Expose of Government Machinations during the Vietnam War.

The Eagle's Feather. A Novel of
International Political Intrigue.

Although The Eagle's Feather is a work of fiction set in the 1970's, it is built, as with most fiction, on a framework of plausibility and background information. This is a fiction book that could not have been written were it not for various ominous aspects, which pose a clear and present danger to the security of the United States.

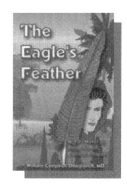

Rhino Publishing

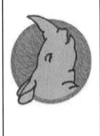

ORDER FORM

PURCHASER INFORMATION

Purchaser's Name (Please Print): _____

Shipping Address (Do not use a P.O. Box): _____

City: _____ State/Prov.: _____ Country: _____

Zip/Postal Code: _____ Telephone No.: _____ Fax No.: _____

E-Mail Address (if interested in receiving free e-Books when available): _____

CREDIT CARD INFO (CIRCLE ONE):

MASTERCARD, VISA, AMERICAN EXPRESS, DISCOVER, JCB, DINER'S CLUB, CARTE BLANCHE.

Charge my Card -> Number #: _____ Exp.: _____

*Security Code: _____ * Required for all MasterCard, Visa and American Express purchases. For your security, we require that you enter your card's verification number. The verification number is also called a CCV number. This code is the 3 digits farthest right in the signature field on the back of your VISA/MC, or the 4 digits to the right on the front of your American Express card. Your credit card statement will show **a different name than Rhino Publishing** as the vendor.

WE DO NOT share your private information, we use 3rd party credit card processing service to process your order only.

ADDITIONAL INFORMATION

If your shipping address is not the same as your credit card billing address, please indicate your card billing address here.

Name on the card _____   Type of card: _____

Billing Address: _____

City: _____   State/Prov.: _____   Zip/Postal Code: _____

Fax a copy of this order to:
RHINO PUBLISHING, S.A.

1-888-317-6767 or International #: + 416-352-5126

To order by mail, send your payment by first class mail only to the following address. Please include a copy of this order form. Make your check or bank drafts (NO postal money order) payable to RHINO PUBLISHING, S.A. and mail to:

Rhino Publishing, S.A.
Attention: PTY 5048
P.O. Box 025724
Miami, FL.
USA 33102

Digital E-books also available online: www.rhinopublish.com

Rhino Publishing

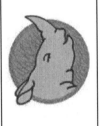

ORDER FORM

Purchaser's Name (Please Print): _____

I would like to order the following paperback book of Dr. Douglass (Alternative Medicine Books):

X ___	9962-636-04-3	Add 10 Years to Your Life. With some "best of" Dr. Douglass writings.	$13.99 $___
X ___	9962-636-07-8	AIDS and Biological Warfare. What They Are Not Telling You!	$17.99 $___
X ___	9962-636-09-4	Bad Medicine. How Individuals Get Killed By Bad Medicine.	$11.99 $___
X ___	9962-636-10-8	Color Me Healthy. The Healing Power of Colors.	$11.99 $___
X ___	9962-636 -XX-X	Color Filters for Color Me Healthy. 11 Basic Roscolene Filters for Lamps.	$21.89 $___
X ___	9962-636-15-9	Dangerous Legal Drugs. The Poisons in Your Medicine Chest.	$13.99 $___
X ___	9962-636-18-3	Dr. Douglass' Complete Guide to Better Vision. Improve eyesight naturally.	$11.99 $___
X ___	9962-636-19-1	Eat Your Cholesterol! How to Live off the Fat of the Land and Feel Great.	$11.99 $___
X ___	9962-636-12-4	Grandma Bell's A To Z Guide To Healing. Her Kitchen Cabinet Cures.	$14.99 $___
X ___	9962-636-22-1	Hormone Replacement Therapies. Astonishing Results For Men & Women	$11.99 $___
X ___	9962-636-25-6	Hydrogen Peroxide: One of the Most Underused Medical Miracle.	$15.99 $___
X ___	9962-636-27-2	Into the Light. New Edition with Blood Irradiation Instrument Instructions.	$19.99 $___
X ___	9962-636-54-X	Milk Book. The Classic on the Nutrition of Milk and How to Benefit from it.	$17.99 $___

___ X	9962-636-00-0	Painful Dilemma - Patients in Pain - People in Prison.	$17.99 $ ___
___ X	9962-636-32-9	Prostate Problems. Safe, Simple, Effective Relief for Men over 50.	$11.99 $ ___
___ X	9962-636-34-5	St. Petersburg Nights. Enlightening Story of Life and Science in Russia.	$17.99 $ ___
___ X	9962-636-37-X	Stop Aging or Slow the Process. Exercise With Oxygen Therapy Can Help.	$11.99 $ ___
___ X	9962-636-60-4	The Hypertension Report. Say Good Bye to High Blood Pressure.	$11.99 $ ___
___ X	9962-636-48-5	The Joy of Mature Sex and How to Be a Better Lover...	$13.99 $ ___
___ X	9962-636-43-4	The Smoker's Paradox: Health Benefits of Tobacco.	$14.99 $ ___

Political Books:

___ X	9962-636-40-X	The Eagle's Feather. A 70's Novel of International Political Intrigue.	$15.99 $ ___
___ X	9962-636-46-9	The W. C. D. Letters. Expose of Government Machinations (Vietnam War).	$11.99 $ ___
		SUB-TOTAL:	$ ___

___	ADD $5.00 HANDLING FOR YOUR ORDER:	$ 5.00 $ 5.00
___ X	ADD $2.50 SHIPPING FOR EACH ITEM ON ORDER:	$ 2.50 $ ___
	NOTE THAT THE MINIMUM SHIPPING AND HANDLING IS $7.50 FOR 1 BOOK ($5.00 + $2.50)	
	For order shipped outside the US, add $5.00 per item	
___ X	ADD $5.00 S. & H. OR EACH ITEM ON ORDER (INTERNATIONAL ORDERS ONLY)	$ 5.00 $ ___
	Allow up to 21 days for delivery (we will call you about back orders if any)	
	TOTAL:	$ ___

Fax a copy of this order to: 1-888-317-6767 or Int'l + 416-352-5126
or mail to: Rhino Publishing, S.A. Attention: PTY 5048 P.O. Box 025724, Miami, FL., 33102 USA
Digital E-books also available online: www.rhinopublish.com

34162905R00052

Made in the USA
Middletown, DE
10 August 2016